BETTER BEING

The go-to guide for healthier choices
from a woman who's made
the mistakes for you

ANN BARNES

Published by Patterns of Behavior, Inc.
Patterns of Behavior, Inc. 600 Bay Street, Suite 200, Toronto, Ontario, Canada, M5G 1M6

This publication contains the opinion and ideas of its author and is designed to provide useful advice in regards to the subject matter covered for information purposes only. This publication is sold with the understanding that neither the author nor the publisher is engaged in rendering health advice or professional services in this publication. The publication is not intended to provide a basis for action in particular circumstances without consideration by a competent professional.

The information contained in this publication cannot replace or substitute for the services of trained professionals in the medical field. You should not act upon any of the information offered or provided within or through this publication without seeking professional advice. In particular, you should regularly consult a doctor in all matters relating to physical or mental health, particularly concerning any symptoms that may require diagnosis or medical attention.

Neither the author nor the publisher make representations or warranties (express or implied) concerning: (i) the information offered or provided within or through the publication; (ii) any treatment, action, or application of medication or preparation by any person following the information offered or provided within or through the publication.

The author and publisher expressly disclaim any responsibility for any liability, loss, risk or damages (consequential, special, exemplary or otherwise), personal or otherwise, that is incurred as a consequence, directly or indirectly, of your reliance on any of the information provided within or through this publication, including but not limited to economic loss, injury, illness or death.

The Library and Archives Canada has cataloged this Patterns of Behavior Publications as follows:
Barnes, Ann
Better Being: A book / by Ann Barnes – 1st ed.

ISBN: 978-0-9865827-0-7

www.beabetterbeing.com

Published and manufactured in Canada.

10   8   7   6   5   4   3   2   1

There are so many people that have been incredible influences but I would specifically like to thank: Mike and Barb Pajak for their continued inspiration, Neil Sheehy from Goodmans LP for being such a brilliant lawyer and mentor, and Vicky for being my health muse. I would also like to thank my family: Dad for his creative and academic brilliance, Mom for acting like an angel while here and who now is one, Tim and Sherrill for being such wonderful siblings and dear friends, my stepson Jaym who keeps me on my philosophical toes, my two wonderful children who are the shining stars in my life and have an inner beauty that leaves me in constant awe, and lastly Mark, the love of my life, who dishes out honesty and encourages me to be the real me.

Table of Contents

Foreword

Restless sleep, sugar and starch cravings, dependence on caffeine, mental fog, difficulty losing fat and developing muscle tone despite a regular exercise routine, immense wave of general fatigue in the afternoon: these are common symptoms of stress. Can you relate? Nearly every North American can, to one degree or another. The problem of stress ranges from being a nuisance to being downright debilitating.

While as problematic as these symptoms may be, they in fact serve an important purpose. Each of them is a "red flag," so to speak, informing us that our body has reached its stress threshold. That's valuable information. However, just like most North Americans, we mask each of these symptoms – shunning them as minor irritants – therefore allowing the cause to not only remain, but to gather momentum and continue to advance. Just as putting a piece of tape over a lit oil light on the dashboard when driving hides the warning light, you no longer have to be immediately aware of the problem. But what caused the light to illuminate continues wreaking havoc that will get worse exponentially and prove costly down the road. And when dealing with humans, not cars, the result can be life-altering.

We drink coffee when fatigued, go on restrictive diets when overweight, and take sleeping pills when we can't sleep. This symptom-treating approach allows the cause to not only remain, but to flourish while veiled.

As I found when researching *The Thrive Diet*, an overwhelming percentage of the average North American's total stress – up to 40 per cent – can be attributed to poor nutrition. We eat foods with very little sustenance – refined and processed – which the body perceives as stressful, since it needs nutrients to burn as fuel and to aid in repair. And as a result, the seemingly strange paradox of being overfed yet undernourished unfolds and becomes the rule, not the exception. And the risk factors of diseases like type 2 diabetes, osteoporosis, cardiovascular disease and arthritis swell considerably. Even several types of cancer can be linked to nutritional shortcomings.

Initially, I found these findings to be disheartening. The fact that our diet was the root cause of our society's rapid health decline didn't sit well with me.

But then it dawned on me – this was good. In fact, it was the best possible situation. Obviously we all control what we eat; therefore, we all have considerable power over our health. We can take charge of our condition and significantly enhance vitality simply by making informed nutritional decisions. And in doing so, we can cut our risk of disease and notably boost our quality of living.

This is where *Better Being* comes in. Taking an approachable manner, Ann not only provides vital information, she shows you how to apply it for lasting results. *Better Being* is a concise, witty handbook written with the sole purpose of enabling you to take charge of your health. Be the exception. Be a Better Being.

Yours in progress,

Brendan Brazier

Preface

Some people change when they see the light,
others when they feel the heat.
Caroline Schroeder, German-American pianist (1882-1952)

The last ten years have had a huge impact on how I live my life. Unlike my mixed-up past, I now lead a happy, relatively clean and healthy existence.

I have finally figured out how to be a good vegetarian in order to properly and easily get the nutrients I need with a plant-based, protein-rich diet. Gone are the days of battling anemia. The vegetarian lifestyle is now a lot easier due to accessible information on its nutritional benefits and the tasty means of living it. Also, let's face it, being a veg is more socially-acceptable now and there are terrific food options.

My struggle with maintaining a healthy body image remains, but to a far lesser degree than the prior years of anorexia and penalty eating. My childhood memories of being overweight and ridiculed have been replaced by the knowledge, power and acceptance that I can create a new and improved version of me by letting go of the negative ghosts of the past. I am further empowered by actively educating myself about the long-term benefits of healthy eating and positive thinking, leaving emotional bingeing and poor nutrition by the wayside.

I am now better equipped to use such knowledge and apply it to how I cook and prepare foods. Food is my passion and always has been, which can be traced back to my early part-time job of catering for film sets. I now apply my love of food to my new-found passion for health and my desire to help those around me learn about and experience the benefits.

My prior fast-paced, stressful life as a corporate and entertainment lawyer, combined with my current chaotic and loving world as a working mother of two young children, has taught me the need for balancing my body, mind and roles (parent, wife, career person, etc.). I know now that without such balance, the whole house of cards can, and will likely, fall. I also now understand the need for healthy food on the go with practical practices that can be easily incorporated into a hectic schedule for both me and my loved ones.

My (and my husband's) experience working with various farmers while owning and operating our natural health food companies, along with our own organic lifestyle on our newly-purchased 100-acre farm, has taught me the vital importance of where food comes from, how it is grown and how it is processed; maintaining high agronomic standards ensures the wholesome nature of the raw ingredients is not compromised. These fundamentals are essential aspects of any food's nutritional composition and potential benefit.

Through all these experiences I have learned so much and I am so grateful. But my current lifestyle and state of mind have not always been this informed or balanced. One of my major turning points for change occurred one early morning many years ago.

It all started in the bathroom.

I knew something was wrong when I faintly heard a familiar man's voice angrily calling my name and realized my cheek was up against a hard cold surface. It was a tiled floor. My bathroom floor. Suddenly aware of the bright light that had just been turned on, I slowly opened my eyes and looked into my husband's irate face.

I slowly raised my torso. My head was pounding. I looked down and realized that I was still in my designer suit and sky-high heels. "What time is it?" I asked, passively aggressively trying to gauge how long I had been sleeping on the floor. "It is 7 a.m., Ann, and you have been lying here since you got home – sometime after three," my hubby angrily informed me. "You have a problem," he announced as he slammed the bathroom door and stormed off to get prepped for another day at his big-whig corporate law firm.

After dusting myself off and scrubbing the stench of scotch off my tongue, I groggily reflected on the previous night's events which had resulted in this matrimonial mess. It started at the city centre's Four Seasons Hotel in a swanky private dining room. I, along with other Toronto and New York lawyers and investment bankers, were celebrating a recently closed $750-million dollar New York deal from a few weeks earlier. Toronto Symphony musicians played while we drank champagne, nibbled on caviar and talked about the financial markets.

After a six course meal, each coupled with a sommelier's choice of wine, the thirty-and-under crowd decided to hit a trendy bar next door. The revelers consisted of me as the only corporate lawyer, along with five New York male investment bankers. At the time, we thought it seemed like a good idea to attempt to sample every brand of scotch the bar offered. The arrogant, young and preppy privileged bankers were new to scotch, but I luckily wasn't.

The bill got paid by someone making a lot more money than me, we were kicked out for overstaying our welcome and I got a taxi home to have a heart-to-heart with the lavatory floor. Upon reflection, I thought, yes, the optics did look bad from hubby's perspective, but I had really done nothing wrong. Right?

My next goal was to get through the day. I showered, brushed my tongue a second time, changed suits, did my hair and proudly got out the door. "My eye hurts," I thought as I sauntered into the lobby of the upscale international insurance company for which I worked. I was one of their many in-house corporate legal counsels. I couldn't believe I had made it in and on time. Perfect!

My assistant brought me my ritual chocolate milk and greasy muffin, which she knew was protocol when I had been "out" the night before. As she brought it to my desk she noted that my right eye was unusually red. All I needed was to look like some pink-eyed party animal in front of my boss. He had attended the previous night's soiree and was sure to ask about the après event. I went to the restroom and realized I had a crisis - my right eye looked like a bulging Japanese flag.

By 10:30 a.m., my eye was swollen shut and the numerous assistants and lawyers on my floor collectively agreed I should go to the hospital. Shamed that my miraculous workplace appearance was now a circus act, I agreed to go. As I threw on my bright red suede coat, I announced that I would return shortly, as I was sure it was really nothing.

The closest hospital was a five-minute walk. Five minutes for both me and most of the city's prostitutes and pimps. As I waited in emergency, I tried desperately to avoid any one-eyed contact with the downtrodden drunks and drug addicts surrounding me. Frustrated at the long wait, I eventually demanded treatment at the emergency admittance station as unlike anyone else there, I had to get back to work. It was then that I turned around to stare into a candy striper's face: it was an old high school friend with whom I had lost touch. "What are you doing here?" she asked. Before I could answer, she blurted out, "God, you reek of booze and you look like hell."

Luckily, she fast tracked me for treatment. I was told I had scratched up my eye pretty badly. My dog's hair had likely found a resting place on my eyeball during my drunken slumber. I was told that I required an eye patch for a few days. "I need to start cleaning my bathroom better," I thought.

Looking like a jazzed up version of Captain Hook, I left the emergency department feeling embarrassed and exhausted. Knowing I was feeling pretty low, my friend took a break and we went to the hospital cafeteria for a late lunch. By then every smell was making me feel sick to my stomach. I had gone through enough.

Over my second greasy muffin of the day, she asked me what I was doing. She asked about my marriage. She asked about my job. She asked why I was out so late, drinking so much. Choking on my stale ball of disguised cake, I started to cry. Then I blurted out the words: "I am so unhappy." Now, once these fateful words are said, you can never go back.

But how did I get to be so unhappy? I had attained my lifelong goal of becoming a lawyer and had experience working at excellent law firms and at a premium company. I married another up-and-coming lawyer with a great family. I had fabulous clothes and a career that looked promising, considering I was only two years in. So why wasn't I appreciative? Why did I feel like I was living outside of my skin?

I realized at that very moment how truly miserable I was. I wasn't in love with my husband. We were great friends, but we should have never taken the plunge. I despised my job and being a lawyer was not what I expected. Instead, I distracted myself with expensive clothing, trendy handbags and "things." I lived a pathetic superficial existence.

After years of dreaming of and working towards the financial security of becoming a corporate lawyer, I knew it made me wretched. But like any well-trained Brownie, I had taken the pledge and I was going to march on with determination to make something of myself. I convinced myself that even if I was unhappy – so what? I would make lots of money, be content as a double-income-no-kids (DINK) family, live in a big downtown house, own lots of designer clothes and drive a spiffy Euro car. Misery is all relative. Or so I thought.

You are now asking yourself: what happened to this uptight, shallow and career-obsessed maniac? Well, after that fateful day and within ten years, I quit my prior life and opted for a new one. I separated from my life of law and got a divorce from the "bathroom man." I met the love of my life with whom I have two beautiful children and became a stepmother to a smart and dynamic teenager. Together my love and I built and ran two health food businesses. We sold off all our worldly goods; okay, not everything, but we got rid of the cottage, two boats, a car, and the city century home. As hard as it was, I even gave away most of my designer clothes. Our nanny was let go and the kids were taken out of their private schools. Substantially lighter in spirit and luggage, we moved to a remote 100-acre farm to practice organic farming and get back to basics. I can't believe I now proudly wear red rubber boots, drive an ATV and stack firewood. And you know what? Life is pretty great.

The reason I am telling you all this is that in my own life journey I have made many mistakes that I repeated over and over again. If I had known then what I now know, my path could have been a lot easier and simpler. In retrospect, I wish I had listened to my inner voice and instincts. I wish I had not been so afraid of change, as my fear prevented me from finding the happiness and balance that was always right in front of me. I also think my changes had to be drastic, since I had so clearly gone down so many wrong paths.

But the radical changes were not made overnight. There was a definite delay between the time I realized my unhappiness with myself and my life and the point when I had the courage to take action to change. Although it did not happen all at once, when I started taking small steps towards change I gained the confidence to make even more. As the power of change kept building, it allowed me to take more substantial action. These larger steps appeared extreme to some but felt quite natural to me once made.

Now that I am at this stage, I look back and realize that in the process of making the "mistakes," I learned so much. Although I wish I could take back my destructive behavior and choices, I also believe nothing is a mistake if you learn from it. One of the best lessons I learned is that wisdom cannot be bought. Wisdom is earned by experience and becomes a wonderful source of knowledge when shared and I am thankful to all who have shared with me.

In turn, I am grateful to have this opportunity to share some of my experiences with you in the hope that you question if and how it relates to you and feel encouraged to make small and easy changes in your life to become a healthier and happier being. Slowly but surely.

Introduction

. . . .

When fire is cried and danger is neigh, "God and the firemen" is
the people's cry; But when 'tis out and all things righted, God is forgotten
and the firemen slighted.
Author unknown, from The Fireman's Journal, England (1879)

I have a lot of respect for firefighters: they are courageous, heroic, physically fit and have incredible stamina and yes, the men are usually not hard to look at. The first time firefighters ever attended my home was when I was at university. There were three of us girls living in a rented house and we all considered ourselves to be bright future stars. One evening, our basement became filled with smoke and we saw flames flickering out of the corner of the dryer. After a frantic call to 911, the firefighters burst through our front door, asked us politely to step aside and quickly put out what little flames there were. After checking thoroughly through the house for any other signs of trouble, the Chief took the three of us aside. He told us, with just a touch of condescension, that the fire was a direct result of not cleaning out the dryer's lint catcher. Our straight-A stars were quite a bit dimmer that evening.

A similar event occurred a few months later. I was driving on the highway in a winter storm and my car just suddenly stopped moving. My used jalopy of a K-car (yes, it was a K-car) had been a generous gift from my parents. After having the car towed, my father's mechanic advised him that the engine had blown and had to be replaced. When asked how this happened, his answer was surprisingly simple: there had been no oil in the engine … apparently for months. My father proceeded to use many swear words I had never heard before. The simple reason "I forgot" was not enough to convince him I had made it past the evolutionary stage of Neanderthal. It was a bad day.

But the point of these two stories is not to let you in on my love of handsome firefighters or my dad's use of expletives. The point is this: in both scenarios, I did not perform the very simple acts required to maintain the machines. For the dryer, cleaning the lint chamber is not only easy, it is the only thing required to prolong a dryer's life span. For the car, it is commonly known that oil is an integral part of running any motor. My lack of attention to these simple solutions was sheer laziness on my part and could have had even more expensive and potentially devastating effects. Like anything, if you do not take the simple steps to keep something well-maintained, it is only a matter of time before it falls apart. Not only does this principle apply to a dryer and a car's body, but to your physical body as well.

Let's be honest. From a health and wellness perspective, the average North American is falling apart. In just the last 20 years, obesity rates in adults and children in North America have consistently increased, even though the weight loss industry has gone from a cottage industry to a thriving economic force. Weight-related diseases such as type 2 diabetes, heart disease, high blood pressure, osteoarthritis, cancer and gallbladder disease have also dramatically increased.

The World Health Organization's 2009 Global Health Risks report listed the world's top mortality risks as high blood pressure (responsible for 13 per cent of deaths globally), tobacco use (9 per cent), high blood glucose (6 per cent), physical inactivity (6 per cent) and obesity or being overweight (5 per cent). These manageable factors raise the risk of chronic diseases, especially the biggest killers such as heart disease, diabetes and cancer and affect all income groups.

Canada, 1978-2005 (18 or older)	1978 (%)	2004 (%)
Total overweight and obese (BMI ≥ 25)	49	59
Overweight (not obese) (BMI = 25 to 29.99)	35	36
Obese (BMI ≥ 30)	14	23
Obese Class I (BMI = 30 to 34.9)	10.5	15
Obese Class II (BMI = 35 to 39.9)	2.3	5.1
Obese Class III (severe) (BMI ≥ 40)	0.9	2.7

Overweight and Obesity, by Age: United States, 1960-2004

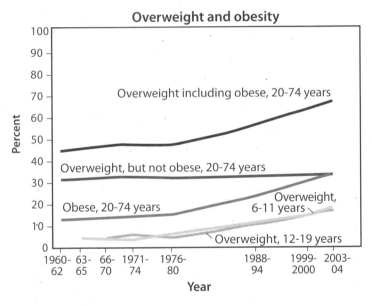

Source: CDC/NCHS, Health, United States, 2006

But why is this happening? With increased accessibility to health-related information, why are we gaining weight at a staggering rate and why are we riddled with preventable diseases? The reality is we have gone from the mode of "upkeep" to "keeping up."

Since the 1950's, we have transitioned from the Rockwellian, Leave-It-to-Beaver lifestyle of our parents and grandparents to the fast-paced materialistic lifestyle we lead today. Advances in technology, coupled with increased commercialism, have come at a major cost. The rise in double-income and single-parent households has resulted in a more frenzied pace than ever, with the continuous rush to and from work and the pressure to find time for family and loved ones, carve out personal time and check off a mile-long list of daily to-dos.

With urban sprawl and mega malls, we spend less and less time at home and far more time in the car – including mealtimes. With our busy schedules and the demand for immediate results, our sit down meals of the past have mutated into food made and delivered to our house by strangers or junk we cram in after cruising through a drive thru. We get take-out in toxic foam containers and buy food from stores in a processed state that is "ready to go" and can be eaten directly out of its package or simply popped in the microwave for that extra sizzle.

Instant gratification is the key to how our culture approaches food and well-being.

- Need to get healthy? Pop some pills.
- Need to downsize that waistline? Do a six-day cleanse or, better yet, staple your stomach – you didn't need that extra lining anyway!
- Have a fat deposit area that just won't give you a break? Just suck it out with your Hoover and then clean the house for good measure!
- Have medical issues? Just self-diagnose yourself online! Why go to a licensed practitioner when you can convince yourself you are dying in front of your living room monitor? Just move to the couch and wait to see the light.

It's all just so... easy.

But is this North American lifestyle all it's cracked up to be? We are so busy going places, but where are we really going? Our reliance on technology for information, education, travel, socialization and entertainment has resulted in a decrease in physical activity. Information bombardment from "interested interest groups," fueled by mega marketing machines, often means that biased information is the first thing we see. In addition, our super-electronic, Facebook-style of community "connectedness" often leaves us feeling alienated and unhealthy.

Because of the frenzied pace at which we function, we develop all kinds of negative eating habits. We overeat as a means to express feelings of loss of control or we develop punitive eating habits (dieting, anorexia, and bulimia) in an attempt to gain back our control. In our age of overstimulation and indulgence, we have created a systemic imbalance in our perception of food and health and how we fit into it all … not to mention how we fit into our jeans!

I'm sure by now you are saying to yourself, "Thanks a lot, Ann. This all sounds so overwhelming. Yes, I know I'm not doing the upkeep on myself that I need and yes, I live in constant information overload and have no time! But I want to improve my health and the health of those I love … so what can I DO?" Well, to put out this wildfire of stress and poor nutrition, we all know the behavioural patterns of the past do not work, so let's look at a new approach that will.

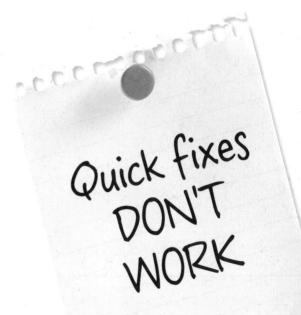

Nurturing the Nurturer

Be a friend to thyself and others will be so too.
Thomas Fuller, English clergyman and historian (1608-1661)

Your body is ultimately all you have: you come into this world with it and it's all you have on the way out. But with the information age in full tilt, the irony is that few people really understand what is required to keep the body properly cared for, to ensure its happiness and longevity. The current quick-fix mentality and express execution cannot work for such a complex structure like the human body. What can we do to bring about changes that will work long term? The answers are surprisingly simple, as it all begins with the way you identify with your body and the level of control you exercise over it.

When we raise kids or own a pet, we do not expect them to grow up overnight. We don't expect a newborn to speak, walk or be able to read and write. We know a teething puppy does not know the difference between the expensive shoes or the dollar store chewy toy. As new parents, we recognize that our child will need a good two to three years (or in my child's case, four years) to become potty trained. We know our pet will need training as well. As a caregiver, we embark upon this process knowing it is a long-term commitment that will require time, energy and a lot of patience to ensure our little rascals, whether furry or not, remain on the right path. We undertake this journey anticipating the need to teach them, train them and nurture them so they develop into the beings we wish them to be, ultimately happy and healthy.

There are really two main approaches to behaviour modification, whether you are dealing with children or puppies: penalty or reward. Either Junior will receive some benefit or reward for good behavior or such benefit or treat is taken away for poor behavior. Having trained four puppies and raised two young children, I can tell you the rewards system works way better.

Why don't we extend the same courtesy to ourselves?

Instead of looking at food as being restrictive or punitive (like diets), if you apply these nurturing principles to yourself, you can learn to provide your body with the proper nutritional upkeep it needs. Over time, you will reach your healthiest potential. Not immediately. Not tomorrow. And probably not by the high school reunion! But know that you can and will get there. Also, you're not the only one who will benefit from good nutrition. Studies show that when parents have good eating habits and nutritional knowledge, their dependants do as well.[3] By better upkeep of yourself, you are also instilling foundational healthy principles for your loved ones.

What does this all mean? It means you need to put your energy into patiently teaching, training and nurturing your mind and body. By understanding how your body works and what effect certain foods have, you can make slight changes to your daily routine to reward yourself and your spirit and see positive long-term results. By following a few simple steps you will start to feel good and, with each passing day, you will get a little bit better and aspire to become the best you can be.

This is my mantra and will hopefully be yours by the end of this book.

To begin, we will get to know how your digestive system works. Next, we will review the three main pillars of nutrients on which your body is built. We will then look at the three main medical challenges facing North Americans when one or more pillars are unbalanced and your building of being becomes lopsided. Lastly, we will look at other ways you can ensure the structure of you remains balanced for optimal well-being with some tasty ways to ensure health and wellness daily.

Three Pillars of Nutrition

. . . .

There is but one temple in the universe and that is the body of man.

Novalis, German poet and philosopher (1772-1801)

Your body is the most incredible and intricate structure on this planet. As complex as it is, it can also be surprisingly simple. The foundation upon which everything rests is made up of the three pillars of major nutrients (macronutrients): fats, carbohydrates and proteins. These three pillars are your energy source, processing and storing energy as it is needed. Your body also needs the smaller nutrients like vitamins and minerals (micronutrients), which rest on top of your pillars in order to make sure your body works to its greatest potential. By keeping your pillars strong and balanced you can build a healthy and productive "Temple of You."

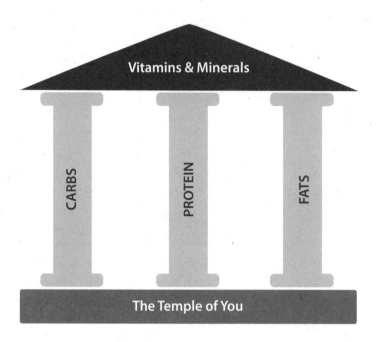

We will review each one of these pillars to understand some basic points you need to know ... and some that will surprise you!

The Ins and Outs

All men by nature desire to know.
Aristotle, Greek philosopher (383 BC – 322 BC)

First of all, to truly understand how the three pillars of nutrition work, you need to understand the ins and outs of your digestive tract. I am just going to give you the nuts and bolts here so things will make more sense when we talk later about what you can do to help your body work better.

The Trash Compactor

When you eat or drink anything, it travels down to your stomach. The stomach breaks down the food into smaller pieces by contracting its layered muscles and releasing acids to kill bacteria and make a mushy mass. If we eat too much, the stomach holds food in the upper bin to be slowly released into the smaller one for later squishing. It releases digestive juices that help separate and break down the carbohydrates, fats and proteins in your food, allowing them to be processed, distributed and stored as body fuel. Once the food is mashed it is then sent on to the small intestine.

The Mail Room

The small intestine is a medical miracle ... forget giving birth! How can 18-20 feet of this intestinal tube all fit so compactly in such a small space? This long pipe acts as the mail room for the partially digested food from the stomach and has three basic functions: (1) it processes the food's nutrients, (2) it helps the nutrients absorb into the bloodstream and (3) it moves the remaining food into the large intestine. Little tiny finger-like tissues in the small intestine sway from side to side to suck up the nutrients and pass them through to your bloodstream or lymph vessels. This amazing feat of nature acts like a bread machine in your insides as it mixes and kneads the food in order to process it. If a toxic substance comes in, this bread machine goes into overdrive to get it out ASAP. (If you've ever had cramps during food poisoning you'll know what I'm talking about.) Whatever liquid or fibre the small intestine cannot absorb is then shipped on to your large intestine for the mass exodus.

The Garbage Dump

The large intestine, also called the bowel or colon, is your body's garbage dump and is made up of two halves that work together. The first half absorbs fluids and recycles them back into your blood stream (where they become the kidneys' problem). The second half compacts the useless junk (feces) and releases a slimy paste to act as a binder and lubricator to ease the downward journey. This stinky mass is mostly water with the rest being undigested food roughage, fat, protein, dried up digestive juices and dead bacteria. Yes, some things I wish I did not know!

The Filtration Plant

The kidneys act as your body's filtration plant. Like a liquid cleanser, they purify your blood and circulate it to the rest of the body. Any toxic fluid waste in the blood is sent from the kidneys to the bladder for storage until you can pee it out. Your kidneys also act as a fluid balancer – if you overeat one day and diet the next your kidneys will level out your fluids, salt and sugar. They are constantly flushing liquids through your system, so drinking a lot of water is key to ensuring they work at their premium. Drink up!

The Nutritional Gatekeeper

The liver also has a lot going on. When you eat, the liver acts as a nutritional gatekeeper – it decides if the food is useful or should be allocated as waste. It also acts as a blood cleanser and detoxifier and can actually alter the chemical composition of toxic substances to make them less harmful to you. It processes nutritional molecules which are eventually distributed to the tissues. From the lungs the liver receives lots of oxygen-rich blood which it sends directly to the heart. It also diverts blood to the intestines to help with digestion and plays an intricate part in producing and storing your body's preferred form of energy (glucose) from sugars, starches and proteins. The liver breaks down cholesterol and fatty acids and produces certain forms of protein needed to clot blood. And if that were not enough, this busy bee also produces a goopy muck called bile, which it sends on to the gallbladder for storage.

The Holding Shed

The gallbladder acts as a holding shed, absorbing mineral salts and water from the liver and stores bile. The bile is then sent to the stomach, which uses it to convert fats to liquids before they are sent to the small intestine.

The Teeter-Totter

Another organ with a huge role (and one we will talk about later in the chapter on diabetes) is the pancreas. It is located on the left side of your body just below your stomach and produces a digestive juice with many enzymes that break down carbohydrates, fat and protein in food. The pancreas also releases hormones that regulate blood sugar levels. It is your body's teeter-totter, helping you maintain a balanced blood sugar level by producing two hormones with opposite actions: insulin and glucagon. Glucagon, released when you are fasting, stimulates your liver and muscles to re-release glucose, making sure your body gets fed and blood sugar levels do not dip too low. Conversely, insulin is released to lower blood sugar levels by stimulating glucose uptake in the blood. It does this by telling the liver and muscle cells to pick up the slack and store the leftover glucose to get it out of your bloodstream. Insulin also stores nutrients for your body by telling the liver and muscle cells to make protein out of the amino acids in foods and tells your fat cells to form fats from fatty acids in foods. It also lets your liver and kidney know when to stop making glucose if it is not needed. The pancreas works hard to ensure your body can maintain a constant and stable blood-glucose level.

As you can see, your digestive system is very complex. Each organ plays a major role that in turn affects another. It is so efficient and intuitive that it allows you to have a wonderful meal out with friends and not even think about all that is going on below. But this feat of nature is also an incredibly sensitive structure. When one area falls apart, the rest will soon follow. Let's find out what you can do to optimize your digestive health and nutritional well-being by effectively using and protecting your three pillars.

The Skinny on Fats

Never eat more than you can lift.
Miss Piggy, celebrity Muppet (b. 1974)

"Fatty, fatty, two-by-four, can't get through the classroom door," was my personal favourite. As a child growing up in a rural farming area, the skinny kids did not hold back. Being the fattest child in my class and a good year younger than the average (as I started school a year early), it certainly wasn't easy. It also didn't help having the last name of Barnes – you can imagine the many opportunities for abusive size-related comments on that one!

I am still not sure to this day if I was overweight due to my British family's high butter and red meat consumption or if it was just my childhood genes gone awry. It is funny to me, especially after having two children, how natural it is to think pudgy rolls on babies are so cute. My poor first-born was poked, prodded and pinched for the first year of his life as he was such a marshmallow. But by about two years old the cuteness of Pillsbury Doughboy bellies and non-existent ankles is suddenly not so adorable and by eight years old it is definitely a source of ridicule. To be clear, by today's supersized standards my then-youthful thigh dimples would be considered nothing more than being "plump." But back then, with kids riding bikes everywhere and a lack of video games to help develop couch potatoes, I was by far the largest kid in my class.

Although the farms were subsequently sold off for subdivisions and my persecutors moved away and spawned skinny children of their own, such painful mockery set me up for two solid decades of an eating disorder, yo-yo dieting and nutrient deprivation. I spent my entire teens and twenties obsessing about how fat (I thought) I was. I measured my knees (yes, I said knees) daily (yes, I said daily). I would place my thumbs together and wrap my hands loosely around each knee. If my index fingers couldn't touch it meant days of deprivation and penalty workouts until they could! My dedication to my knee project would have been the envy of any Girl Guide pounding the pavement to sell her cookies. Unfortunately, my mission was in no way positive.

In my early twenties, my pathetic attempt to gain back a feeling of control over my life manifested itself in trying to break the 100-pound mark. I restricted my calorie intake to fewer than 900 a day – half of what I should have been eating – and ate little if no fat due to my belief that "fat makes you fat." At 5'6", the lowest weight I reached was 102 pounds and at 21 years of age I looked like a scrawny 12-year-old boy. As hard as I tried, I could not lose any more weight. I now know that my body went into shock mode to hold on to anything I fed it for fear it would not eat for a while. My once lovely skin became dry and pimply, my energy level was low and my memory was shot. I was waiting tables at the time and would literally take an order for drinks from a table of two, head into the back to fulfill it and would forget what they had said. Although thin, I was nutritionally starved and it was negatively affecting every aspect of my life.

After years of self-abuse and low self-esteem, I finally turned the corner. It took a pregnancy for me to actually embrace being big. It also forced me to seek out the truth about fats and other aspects of nutrition that before then had been based upon folklore, media misinformation and fashion magazines. What I know now is how important fats are to my body and that it is imperative to get enough of the good ones. To clear up the mystery surrounding it, let's wrestle this fat fable to the ground and find out what fats are, how they work and what foods you can use to ensure you get what your body needs.

Fat – What does it mean?

The word "fat" has a few different meanings. It can mean:

- *Fat cells*, the fatty tissue under your skin and on top of each of your kidneys.
- *Fat molecules*, which are made by your body as a source of stored fuel and which stuff the fat cells (the stuffin' in those love handles).
- *Food fats* you eat such as olive oil, nut oils, butter, etc. These come in a number of forms (unsaturated, saturated or mutated) and have varying levels of nutritional benefits – the good, the bad and the ugly.

Let's go through each one and figure out what you need to know to help you on your journey.

Fat Cells

Now listen to me when I say this: fat cells are your friend! They have an important job to do as they absorb vitamins, control blood pressure and keep you warm. In fact, your brain is made up of 60 per cent fat cells and in young children, developing fat cells are critical for the brain and the immune system.[4] Whether you are male (apple-shaped) or female (pear-shaped) will determine where most of your fat cells are located: which is why women have "thunder thighs" and men have "beer bellies." No one ever grows more fat cells; the ones you have just get stuffed with more fat molecules. An obese man and a cover girl have the same number of fat cells, but, much like balloons, the obese man's are inflated to their maximum size and the model's have yet to be blown up (poor girl!).

Fat Molecules

Fat molecules are made by your body from either the food fat you eat or from the surplus carbohydrates or protein in your diet. Whatever you eat, regardless of what it is, your body immediately uses the calories you are consuming for quick energy. If there are any calories left over that are not needed at that time, two things happen: First, your fat cells absorb the leftover fat molecules (that are made from the food fat). Second, they eventually convert the unused protein and carbs into even more fat molecules. This is why when you consistently overeat on any foods you are essentially stuffing your fat cells with fat molecules and will eventually become big. All fat molecules are stored in your fat cells for future energy use. But fat molecules are not your body's first choice of fuel – carbohydrates are. When you need energy, your body will proceed to use up the carbs first, then the fat molecules. The fat stored literally sticks around until the body has no other choice but to use it (kind of like being the last one picked for the team). Unfair but true.

Food Fats

Food fats are here to stay, which is a good thing as their creamy consistency helps to make our food taste so good! Other than trans fats, which I will get to later, food fats are one of the three major nutritional pillars of your diet. Food fats, like people, come in a number of shapes and sizes. Note that fatty foods are usually made up of a combination of fats with a higher concentration of one specific type. Let's review the three various types of food fat.

Saturated Fat (S-Fat)

These are the scrumptious and creamy, thighs-a-mile-high fats which include animal foods like butter, tallow, lard, cream, meat and cheese and tropical oils such as coconut oil and palm kernel oil. They are the most chemically-stable kind of fat and can withstand the highest cooking temperatures, remaining solid unless heated. When you eat foods that contain S-Fat, your body responds by raising the bad cholesterol levels (LDL) in your blood, which over time can increase your risk of heart disease and stroke. Also, many S-Fat-rich foods (animal-based) are already high in cholesterol, which adds more flame to the bad cholesterol fire. Because of these negative effects, S-Fats should be eaten in limited quantity and frequency, as they are the "bad" fats.

One anomaly to this S-Fat conundrum is non-hydrogenated coconut oil. Although an S-Fat, it has antiviral, antibacterial and antimicrobial properties due to its high levels of lauric acid – one of the most important essential fatty acids (EFAs) in building and maintaining the body's immune system. Although coconut oil is made up of 92 per cent S-Fats, 62 per cent of it is made up of saturated medium chain triglycerides. When three fatty acids bind together they make a triglyceride that also comes in S, M and L, with each size functioning very differently. Most fats consumed by the average North American are long-chain triglycerides, which are hard to digest. But research shows that medium chain fatty acids, as found in coconut oil, help increase your metabolism and are more easily digested as they are processed directly in the liver and are immediately converted into energy. The result? Your liver and pancreas have less strain and your body gets a quick and efficient source of energy. Coconut oil is also less caloric than its S-Fat counterparts such as butter and lard, making coconut oil a "good" S-Fat because it acts more like a carbohydrate than a fat.

Polyunsaturated Fat (P-Fat)

Foods high in P-Fat include corn oil, safflower oil, walnut oil, fish oils, oily fish (herring, salmon, mackerel and halibut), grains, and eggs. They are the most unstable of all food fats, as in their oil state, these fats can go rancid when exposed to sunlight, air or heat. P-Fat-based oils are best used in their raw form and kept in the fridge, so pay close attention to expiration dates. Some research suggests that too much P-Fat can increase the risk of cancer and the incidences of tumors.[5] But they can also help reduce the cholesterol levels in your blood and lower your risk of heart disease.

P-Fat is also the only food fat with the two essential fatty acids: omega-6 fatty acids as found in hemp seed, hemp oil, avocado, nuts, evening primrose oil, borage oil, blackcurrant seed oil, eggs, pumpkin seeds, safflower oil, corn oil, sesame oil and sunflower oils; and omega-3 fatty acids as found in Salba (Salvia hispanica L), cold-water oily fish, linseed oil, camelina seeds, hemp seeds, hemp oil and walnuts. These EFA-specific types of P-Fat are the very, very "good" fats.

Essential fatty acids, or EFAs, are just that: ESSENTIAL! These cannot be made by your body so you need to get them from your food. The average North American does not get anywhere near the amount of omega-3's that is needed. Studies show that EFAs are vital for growth and maintencance of cells, and some can provide greater energy, increase brain function, improve skin quality, decrease blood pressure and make your blood less likely to clot. EFAs are truly one of the easiest things to add to your daily routine to get the most bang for your buck!

The optimum balance between these two EFAs in our diet is considered to be a 1:1 ratio, which contrasts with the current balance of about 20:1 in the average Western diet. The high omega-6 ratio is thought to be directly linked North American's high consumption of corn and sunflower oils in processed foods which can lead to chronic inflammation. To balance this, omega-3 consumption is instrumental in balancing the dietary imbalance. Also, one important omega-6 that can assist your body is gamma-linolenic acid (GLA) as found in mother's milk, hemp seeds, hemp oil, borage oil and evening primrose oil. Unlike some other omega-6's, GLA has anti-inflammatory properties and has been researched for asthma management and treating skin disorders and certain cancers.[6]

EFAs play a vital role in overall health as they slow down fat production and increase energy, which in turn burns more calories. Conversely, an EFA deficiency has been associated with cardiovascular disease, cancer, diabetes and other degenerative conditions which are accountable for over 60 per cent of deaths in North America. Symptoms of EFA-deficiency include diarrhea, inflammation of joints, dandruff, dry skin, hair loss, brittle nails, immune impairment, infertility, poor wound healing, yeast/ Candida infection, premenstrual syndrome, dry eyes/mouth/throat and excessive ear wax.

Monounsaturated Fat (M-Fat)

M-Fat-rich foods include vegetable oils such as olive oil, canola oil, peanut oil, sunflower oil and sesame oil and foods such as avocados, nuts and seeds. M-Fat oils remain liquid at room temperature but can become semi-solid or solid when refrigerated. High use of olive oil in Mediterranean diets is considered to be one of the reasons why those countries have substantially lower levels of heart disease. This is because M-Fat helps reduce bad cholesterol levels in your blood and can lower your risk of heart disease and stroke. M-Fat is also typically high in vitamin E, which is a known antioxidant, making it another "good" fat.

Trans Fatty Acids (TFAs)

Trans fatty acids lurk in delectably-mouthwatering greasy foods, tempting us until we succumb to their evil ways. Other than small amounts naturally occurring in some dairy products and cow and sheep meat, these delicious demons are not found in nature and are not natural to our bodies. They are man-made fats found in partially hydrogenated vegetable oils. Through a chemical process, the vegetable M-Fats and P-Fats are chemically and physically altered by injecting hydrogen into them under high pressure and heat, which makes them high in trans fatty acids. They are like newly mutated fat zombies. As they are absorbed into our bodies, they lower good cholesterol (HDL) and raise the bad cholesterol (LDL).[7] The end result is that consumption of TFAs increases cholesterol levels in our blood, which can lead to a number of illnesses that we will discuss later.

Additionally, as TFAs cannot be easily absorbed into our bodies, the enzymes needed to break them down cannot effectively process the good-for-you EFAs. TFAs are like the bad kid in the classroom who monopolizes the teacher's time, which means the well-behaved kids don't learn as much as they could.

So why does the food industry make and use these cholesterol-ridden mutants? The sole purpose of such hydrogenation is to extend the shelf stability of the oil products and to reduce costs, as it is a cheap substitute for the better-for-you fats. Unfortunately, many grocery and restaurant pre-packaged or frozen foodshave them such as: prepared baked goods, cereals, chips, fried foods, cake mixes, ramen noodles, soup cups, dips, salad dressings, breakfast cereals, salty snacks, crackers, cookies, candies, international coffee blends, microwave popcorn, vegetable shortening and some margarines. When shopping, avoid TFAs by scouring the nutritional labels for any foods with ingredients such as partially-hydrogenated vegetable oils, hydrogenated vegetable oils or shortening.

Frying
Another change occurs when you heat any kind of fat. When you are cooking with oil, you have to match the heat tolerance of the oil you are using, as oils at too high a temperature can become carcinogenic. Oils high in P-Fat such as soya, canola, sunflower and corn oils degrade easily to toxic compounds when heated past their smoke point.[8] Also, long-term consumption of burnt oils can lead to atherosclerosis, inflammatory joint disease and the development of birth defects. So if you burn it, throw it out![9]

To reduce the heat of oil, put a small amount of water in the frying pan first, then add oil. This will hydrate the food but also reduce the chance of burning the oil. It is important to know that heat applied to any food, whether a fat or not, will cause enzymes to be destroyed, proteins to become denatured and vitamins and minerals to become less available. The less heat or frying, the better! No heat or frying is best.

The following chart of smoke points (the maximum temperature to which you should heat various oils) is helpful and healthful.[10]

Fat	Smoke Point °F	Smoke Point °C
Unrefined canola oil	225°F	107°C
Unrefined flaxseed oil	225°F	107°C
Unrefined safflower oil	225°F	107°C
Unrefined sunflower oil	225°F	107°C
Unrefined corn oil	320°F	160°C
Unrefined high-oleic sunflower oil	320°F	160°C
Extra virgin olive oil	320°F	160°C
Unrefined peanut oil	320°F	160°C
Semirefined safflower oil	320°F	160°C
Unrefined soy oil	320°F	160°C
Unrefined walnut oil	320°F	160°C
Hemp seed oil	330°F	165°C
Butter	350°F	177°C
Semirefined canola oil	350°F	177°C
Coconut oil	350°F	177°C
Unrefined sesame oil	350°F	177°C
Semirefined soy oil	350°F	177°C
Vegetable shortening	360°F	182°C
Lard	370°F	182°C
Refined canola oil	400°F	204°C
Semirefined walnut oil	400°F	204°C
High quality (low acidity) extra virgin olive oil	405°F	207°C
Sesame oil	410°F	210°C
Cottonseed oil	420°F	216°C
Grapeseed oil	420°F	216°C
Virgin olive oil	420°F	216°C
Almond oil	420°F	216°C
Hazelnut oil	430°F	221°C
Peanut oil	440°F	227°C
Sunflower oil	440°F	227°C
Refined corn oil	450°F	232°C
Refined high-oleic sunflower oil	450°F	232°C
Refined peanut oil	450°F	232°C
Refined safflower oil	450°F	232°C

Summary

Our body needs fat to properly function, especially the good fats such as EFAs and the cholesterol-reducing M-Fats. Excluding coconut oil, the S-Fats are not so great and the TFAs are downright evil. But if you are eating too much of any food in comparison with the energy you are using, your fat cells will stuff themselves with fat molecules, resulting in a bigger you. But the reality is this: you are the one allowing your fat cells to become stuffed. If you stop and listen to your body and ask yourself, "Am I still really hungry?" or "How is this fat making me feel right now?" you may be surprised at your body's answer.

Also remember that no matter which fat you chose to eat, all fats, no matter how healthy, are high in calories: each gram of fat has nine calories. When compared to the svelte four calories per gram of carbohydrate or protein, fats have more than twice as much. Increase your intake of the healthy fats and dump the unhealthy ones, with a goal of having between 15- 25 per cent of your daily calories coming from any fat source. So get the good ones in!

What you know now:
- Fat cells are your friend! They help absorb vitamins, control blood pressure and keep you warm.
- You need to have good fat daily; aim to get in no more than 25 per cent of your daily calories from good fat sources.
- Choose the best fats based upon the following:
  - Trans Fatty Acids = TFAs = The Fats to Avoid
  - Saturated Fat = S-Fat = Sometimes
  - Polyunsaturated Fat = P-Fat = Pick Carefully (an EFA)
  - Essential Fatty Acids= EFAs = Essential For All!
  - Monounsaturated Fat = M-Fat = Most of the Time
- Avoid fried foods and try not to fry, but if you must ... not so hot!

Apply to your daily routine:
- When grocery shopping:
  - Avoid foods with "partially-hydrogenated," "hydrogenated" or "shortening" listed on the label.
  - Make better fat choices of M-Fat and P-Fat (EFAs!!!)

- Sneaky tip: if the TFA is not listed, then add up the P-Fat, S-Fat and M-Fat. Subtract this number from the total fat listed and this is your TFA amount.
- When cooking or out at a restaurant, opt for dishes that are grilled, steamed or baked rather than fried.
- When frying, start with a small amount of water in the pan and then add your oil or fat. To fry, use healthy oil that maintains a higher smoke point, like olive oil, sesame or avocado oil.
- Eat EFA-rich foods daily by adding Salba seeds to your cereals or yogurt in the morning, hemp seeds or hemp oil to your salads, salad dressings, soups or stews and if you eat fish opt for low-mercury unfarmed oily fish for meals.
- Substitute coconut oil for butter or margarine in baking recipes (¾ cup coconut oil to 1 cup shortening) for a good S-Fat option or substitute up to ¾ of the shortening in the recipe with unsweetened applesauce.

Carbohydrates: How Sweet It Is

When my horse is running good, I don't stop to give him sugar.
Douglas Horton, clergyman and Harvard academic (1891 – 1968)

I am convinced lawyers don't have bowel movements. Nor do corporate executives. In my ten-year legal career, nobody I worked with ever spoke of having one: not in the exclusive law firms located in the skyscrapers of Toronto's financial district, nor in the numerous corporate legal departments in which I found myself.

During long and often tedious meetings, you never admitted where you were actually going when excusing yourself. Of course, the reason for excusing yourself was usually due to the five cups of coffee sucked back in an attempt to stay awake. The only time anyone came close to admitting to "human elimination abilities" was when select men in the elite law firms would hastily grab the financial sections of newspapers from the glass lobby tables on their way to the restroom. Everyone knew what they were up to. Trust me – I will never touch another newspaper in a corporate lobby again. Apparently, lawyers and executives do not urinate and they do not have bowel movements. They must be stuffed full of it, which could explain a lot!

Fast forward to the world I chose when I left my life of law and entered the health food industry. Owning and operating a healthy food company with my husband allowed me to meet many people at food shows, in stores and over the phone. My newfound life allowed for free flow discussions on healthy living, which prevailed over my previous and tedious cocktail conversations on the merits of Shareholders' Rights Agreements.

What was initially shocking to me on my new path of health and honesty was how willing people are to discuss their very personal experiences in the restroom. What I found even more surprising was how many people admitted to suffering from long-term problems with their bowel movements. The majority of people I spoke with had one every couple of days, but those with the worst stories had only one every five or six days! Now, if you think of how your body works, your food provides your body with energy that is used right away or stored for later use. What it intuitively knows it does not need is then shipped off to the throne. When this refuse is not expelled, but instead remains in your intestinal tract, you are basically being stuffed with ... well, crap. This waste literally gets stuck to your intestinal walls and is hard to unglue once lodged. What is worse is that because all major organs are attached to your intestines, the toxic garbage can seep back into other organs and your blood stream. And we wonder why North Americans are so sick?

One of the major means of getting your body back to the input/output schedule it needs is for you to understand carbohydrates and the huge benefits of fibre, as these are the main ingredients in allowing your inner septic system to "go with the flow."

The Misunderstood Carbohydrate

Carbohydrates (carbs) are naturally occurring in many foods we eat – like cereals, grains, fruits and vegetables – but are sadly misunderstood. So many people restrict their consumption of carbs as a means of weight loss. (Recall the popular low-carb diets?) But carbs are actually your body's preferred energy source because they are easiest for your body to use.

Carbs allow for the proper functioning of the kidneys, central nervous system and muscles, including your heart. Importantly, carbs are the only source of energy used by the brain. Carbs are either used right away or stored in your muscles and liver for future use and they play an integral role in ensuring a healthy intestine and efficient waste elimination. Too few carbs can result in fatigue, poor brainpower and the breakdown of muscle tissue and can manifest in physical symptoms such as nausea, weakness, dizziness and mood swings.

Carbs come in two sizes: the simple small ones and the complex big ones.

Simple Carbs (S-Carbs)

S-Carbs are small molecules of sugar: glucose, fructose and galactose. As they are small and easy to digest, your body quickly absorbs them. If your body doesn't need that high level of energy right then and there, then the simple sugars will quickly be converted for future energy storage either in your cells or, if the cells are maxed out, as fat. This is why foods high in sugar are often referred to as "empty" calories, as there isn't much benefit to them other than that minute on the lips. S-Carbs hang out in those mouthwatering temptations such as cakes, pastries and other baked goods, biscuits, candies and table sugar. Your blood sugar raises and spikes quickly when you eat these empty S-Carb calories with no nutritional benefits. In a desperate attempt to regulate this spike, your pancreas quickly responds and secretes insulin to regain balance. A diet rich in these tasty airheads results in pressure on your pancreas, which eventually may shut down, and may contribute to a pre-diabetic condition or directly to type 2 diabetes.

Unlike the ooey-gooey baked goods, unprocessed nutrient-rich foods like fruit contain naturally-occurring S-Carbs. However, due to the low levels of the sugar in the fruit, the body can more easily absorb the sugar, lowering the chance for it to be converted to fat. Also, many fruits are fibre-rich so your digestion is slowed, which allows the natural sugars to be slowly introduced to your body. To sum it up, fruit is an S-Carb that is a wannabe complex carb.

Complex Carbs (C-Carbs)

C-Carbs are simply sugars that like each other and have bonded together to form a Big Momma of a sugar chain. Because they are bigger, your digestive enzymes have to work that much harder to break them down so they can be absorbed through your intestines. This is a slow process which means that your body S-L-O-W-L-Y absorbs the energy and provides it to you in a steady supply, which limits the amount of sugar converted into fat for storage. By maintaining a steady flow of glucose through your blood stream, you will ensure optimal fat burning efficiency and have long-term appetite control with minimal food cravings. C-Carbs are broken down into two types: starch and fibre.

Starch

Starch is naturally produced by all green plants as an energy reserve and is a major food source for humans. Starches are long complex chains of simple sugars. Although a C-Carb, some starches are so quickly absorbed by the body that absorption starts in your mouth! Most starchy foods are rapidly broken down into sugar so people who are sensitive to sugar should avoid most starchy foods as well. Starch-rich foods include: corn, rice, potatoes, beans and all grains (wheat, rice, barley and oats). The bad rap on starch happens when the original whole food is processed into a ground, puffed, flaked or rolled version. Instead of your body doing some of the good work itself, food is immediately delivered in a final form (like flour or processed breakfast cereal) to be quickly turned into sugar in your system. The result of such processing is a spike in your blood sugar levels followed by a low. The good news is that starches that remain in their whole and unprocessed state, like whole grains, legumes, beans, brown rice or whole barley, will allow the sugar to be digested more slowly or not absorbed at all. This is called a resistant starch and is easier on your system.

Fibre

The carbs that cannot be digested are referred to as fibre. Fibre can only be found in plant-related food. Fibre is our body buddy, as it has many benefits: it helps to promote regularity, decreases the risk of heart disease and lowers cholesterol. It can also assist in weight loss and weight management, as it makes you feel full longer. Diets low in fibre can cause problems such as constipation and hemorrhoids and high fibre diets can decrease the risk of certain types of cancer, especially colon cancer.[11] Fibre-rich foods include fruits (with edible skin and seeds) and veggies (especially the leafy greens), oats, barley, buckwheat, coconut, nuts, seeds, kidney beans, lentils, pinto beans, lima beans, navy beans and split peas.

There are two kinds of fibre: soluble (S-Fibre) and insoluble (I-Fibre) and we need both of them – preferably a 1:3 ratio for best digestive health.

S-Fibre binds with fatty acids in your stomach and slows down the absorption rate of glucose in your blood. By doing so, it helps to stabilize your blood sugar levels by reducing the sugar spikes. When you have a sugar high, your pancreas stimulates the production of insulin, which over time can contribute to type 2 diabetes and increase the risk of heart disease and strokes. (More on this in the section "The Three Major Threats.") One of S-Fibre's greatest features is that it attracts water and turns into a gel during digestion. Like a fibrous sponge, it sucks up water and gets heavier as it moves through your system. The heavier the better, as waste is dragged down with it and is quickly processed through the intestines. S-Fibre also helps prevent constipation, as the absorbed water lubricates your tube and can protect against diseases of the colon such as colon cancer and diverticulitis. S-Fibre can also help control your appetite, because the glucose is slowly brought into your system, making you feel full for longer. It is found mainly in fruits, veggies like carrots, barley, oats, beans and lentils.

I-Fibre works in conjunction with S-Fibre to help you maintain a healthy digestive system. The intestinal benefit of I-Fibre is that as it moves though the large intestine, it acts as a kind of internal snow plow which helps to remove toxins and waste, allowing your intestines to absorb more nutrients and produce less harmful bacteria. It also helps to balance intestinal pH levels by reducing your body's acidity. I-Fibre also improves intestinal health by increasing stool volume and stimulating normal bowel contractions, which can help reduce waste transit time. A speedy exodus helps to protect against digestive problems like constipation, diverticulitis and irritable bowel syndrome. Nuts, seeds and whole grains are the main source of I-Fibre.

So how much do you need? Based upon a 1,800-calorie daily diet, it is recommended that 55 per cent of calories come from carbohydrates with 25-35 grams of fibre (depending upon age, sex and weight). In contrast, the average Canadian adult consumes only half of the recommended daily amount![12]

Luckily, it is not too hard to increase your daily fibre intake without a lot of work. Some simple painless steps include:
- Switch from white bread to whole grain bread, which immediately doubles fibre intake. Rememeber that whole grains trump whole wheat and whole wheat trumps white.
- Opt to snack on fruit and nuts instead of chips or chocolate. This will pump you with the fibre you need along with lots of vitamins and protein.
- Beans and brown rice are rich in fibre and together deliver a punch of protein, so use them as an inexpensive meat substitute in soups, stews and casserole dishes.

- Use fibre rich nut butter on toast instead of margarine, butter or jam.
- Anytime something is refined, it strips more nutrients away.
- Choose as much unrefined food as you can.
- For breakfast pick a whole oatmeal cereal or unsweetened granola with nuts rather than preprocessed corn flakes or puffed rice cereals.
- Eat your fruit, don't drink it! That way you get the benefits of all the fibre fruit naturally has to offer.

But remember, treat your body gently. Increase your fibre slowly in small amounts. Add a five gram increase every five days until you reach the 20-35 grams a day mark. If you add fibre too quickly you risk becoming a bloated boom box while waiting for your body to adjust. When increasing fibre intake, always drink more water to help move it down the chute and to remove the toxins!

Summary
Like fats, carbs are often misunderstood. Carbs help the kidneys function better and provide efficient and preferred energy, which is necessary to feed your brain and give you a healthy heart and strong muscles. But, like fat, it is only healthy if you have the RIGHT kind.

One of the easiest ways to understand carbs is to imagine that your body is in a constant marathon race. If you enter a high-speed sprinter (S-Carb) into the race, they will exit the starting line quickly only to fall face down after the first couple of laps. Although starting out slowly, the C-Carb wins the race every time, as it is slow and steady. The next time you are about to bite into a S-Carb cupcake, remember that it's an empty-headed sprinter about to do a huge face plant on your buttocks!

Fibre can also help get rid of the toxic waste in your intestinal tract, which brings us back to our original dilemma of the poor poo passage. It is generally thought that the "rule-of-bum" should be at least one solid bowel movement a day. Always be aware of how your body is flushing itself out, as constipation (fewer than three bowel movements in a week) or diarrhea can indicate a poor diet with too little fibre. If you feel bloated, don't have regular bowel movements or have something other than a gentle S curve result when you do go, your body is sending up smoke signals to tell you there is something you need to change. Give yourself a break and start listening to what your intuitive temple is telling you. If you don't listen when your body whispers, it will soon start to YELL at you!

What you know now:
- Carbs are sugars your body converts into glucose, a fuel your body needs, but not all carbs are considered equal.
- S-Carbs are simple sugars and, other than those found in fruits, they are absorbed quickly, leading to highs and lows in the blood which can be hard on your pancreas and contribute to greater body fat.
- C-Carbs are the ones you must befriend as they are slowly digested. This leaves you feeling full longer and reduces the sugar spikes.
- Fibre is an indigestible C-Carb that helps you have regular bowel movements, stabilizes weight, lowers blood sugar levels and assists in ensuring a healthy heart.
- Irregular bowel movements are a warning sign of bad digestive health or diet. Gently add more fibre to your diet to blow this problem away!

Apply to your daily routine:
- Opt for protein dense whole beans, lentils, brown rice, buckwheat, barley, amaranth or quinoa when choosing starchy foods.
- Give up the baked goods or flour-based treats unless they are high in fibre.
- Stay full longer by choosing high-fibre foods at each meal of the day.
- Boost fibre slowly until you are averaging 20-35 grams per day and aim for a 1:3 ratio of S-Fibre to I-Fibre.
- Drink lots of water, because your internal waterslide needs it.
- Make small changes by making better food choices and over time it will have a huge impact. Remember that for rice and bread brown is better and white is wasted!
- Combine S-Carbs with S-Fibre to slow down digestion and decrease those sugar spikes.
- Avoid processed starchy foods especially at breakfast, whether ground, puffed, or flaked.
- Get your veggies every day – they're a great source of low-cal, high-fibre carbs.

Protein Power

More die in the United States of too much food than of too little.
J.K. Galbraith, American economist (1908-2006)

I blame my mother's bad cooking for the reason I became a vegetarian. God rest her soul, but there were two settings for our oven: 400 degrees or broil. I cannot ever recall seeing a roast beef that wasn't the colour of mud or the consistency of shoe leather. Not even dousing it in a pool of gravy could soften that baby up. However, I do have to thank my mom for my strong teeth, as my back molars were broken in on her Sunday night dinners.

I decided to give up meat the day I saw the tongue. I was about 13 years old and was walking through the kitchen when I spotted it. Sitting upright on a pan was the whole tongue of a cow, looking like a silent scream without lips. Now, I had eaten tongue before but only as a sliced up pile of brown mass on a plate. It had never occurred to me prior to this moment that what I was eating was a real-life tongue. It was like a Rolling Stone album cover but only so much more authentic. My mom had worked her usual culinary skills and had spread about half a pound of butter over the speechless thing and sprinkled some pepper and paprika over it for good measure. The tongue visual traumatized me for a very long time and set me up for a life of vegetarianism.

When I left home some five years later, I was finally able to be the aspiring vegetarian I had envisioned. No more meat! I also decided this did not go far enough, so I then cut out all dairy, eggs and fish. I now had an impressive title: I was a vegan! I was healthy! I was right! I was ... self-righteous. My well-intentioned plan to become a powerhouse of nutrition as a result of my plant-based diet quickly slipped into nutritional deprivation. Basing my vegan life around raw carrots and white rice with a couple of dill pickles thrown in for salty goodness left me feeling lethargic and iron deficient. Vanity kicked in when I realized I had horrible skin coupled with a highly unattractive orange glow. Like many "bad" vegetarians, I was protein deficient.

Of the three pillars of nutrition, protein is by far the most understood by the average person. But did you know that proteins make up every cell, tissue and organ in your body? Proteins help build, maintain and replace the tissue required for your muscles, organs, bones and immune system.

There are thousands of different types of proteins with various combinations, each made up of protein building blocks called amino acids. When you eat protein-rich foods, the amino acids are singularly broken down in your stomach and intestines and are then recycled back into your system to make the specific proteins your body needs to maintain itself. For example, protein is used to make the red blood cells that carry oxygen all over your body and is also used to build muscle (most importantly, your heart!). Of the protein building blocks, there are 22 amino acids in total. Your body can only make 14 of them and the remaining 8 (called essential amino acids (EAAs)) have to be obtained solely by foods. So where can you get them?

EAAs are found in both animal and vegetable sources. When a food has all 22 amino acids, including EAAs, it is called a complete protein. Complete proteins are available in animal foods such as meat, fish, eggs and dairy products like milk, yogurt and cheese. Amaranth, blue-green algae, buckwheat, hemp seed, Salba seeds, soybeans, quinoa and spirulina are the only plant-based foods with all 22 EAAs you need. Complete proteins are the "no-brainers" to eat as you don't have to think about sourcing any other amino acids. Other vegetable-based proteins are incomplete because they lack one or more of the EAAs. These include nuts, seeds, grains, legumes and beans.

But, like any good fashionista, proteins can be mixed and matched for a rich experience. You can still get all your EAAs by eating a wide variety of protein-rich vegetable foods. By mixing beans, lentils or peas with nuts, seeds or whole grains, the proteins combine to have a Tom Cruise moment – they complete each other. By combining beans and rice, or corn and beans, or peanut butter on whole grain bread, you actually make a complete protein. Also, your mixing and matching of amino acids can take place throughout the day because the EAAs don't have to be eaten all at once; just within 24 hours.

Although it is good to mix it up a little, it is important to source your protein carefully to get the most bang for your buck. Many of the foods you might think are high in protein may not be such a great choice upon closer review. Like the cute crush that always brings the annoying friend along, avoid the proteins with bad tag-alongs:

Meat

While high in protein, non-lean red meats and processed meats are also high in S-Fat. In a recent study on cancer prevention, researchers suggested the amount of red meat eaten should be limited. In the same study, they suggested processed meats containing sodium nitrate such as bacon, ham, hot dogs, deli meats, smoked fish and corned beef should be completely avoided due to the convincing evidence that eating sodium nitrate increases the risk of colorectal cancer.[13] If you have children, rethink the kid "staples" of hot dogs and pepperoni pizza as they are potentially cancer on bread.

If you eat meat, be sure to select skinless, lean cuts and opt for low-fat dairy products. Also, red or white meat does not contain any fibre making it a pretty limited protein compared to the fibre-rich plant sources available. If you opt for fibre-less meat options, make sure that you also pare it with a fibre-rich side.

Fish

Wild fish may have a better rap, but may also be contaminated with high levels of mercury. Fish harvesting is often very hard on the environment as trawling nets destroy the ocean floor and other ocean life. Fish farms are no better, as they commonly use mulched wild fish pellets to feed the farmed fish, increasing the mercury contamination and/or the damage to the environment. Knowing where and how the fish are harvested and what they consumed are key points in knowing the health benefits or risks of the fish you are eating.

Cow's milk

Cow's milk has a great deal of S-Fat and high calories with a relatively low amount of protein. Better and cheaper protein sources are available with less caloric costs.

Protein Mixes

Most commercially mixed protein powders should be avoided because they often contain artificial sweeteners like aspartame, which is linked to neurological disorders. Other sweeteners are not much better, since they contain no nutritional value and trick your body into thinking it is eating something sweet with possible harmful side effects. If you opt for a protein powder make sure they are clean and green.

Cheese

While delicious, cheese is chock-full of S-Fats and shouldn't be used as a staple source of protein. Use cheese with strong a flavour so less is more.

Instead of the above, good sources of protein can be easily obtained by adding any of the following to your daily meals or snacks:
- 2 tablespoons hemp seed (10g complete protein)
- 2 tablespoons hemp protein powder (13g complete protein)
- 1 cup cooked quinoa (9g complete protein)
- 1 egg (6g complete protein)
- 1 cup low-fat milk (8g complete protein)
- 1 cup low-fat yogurt (11g complete protein)
- 2 tablespoons peanut butter (7g protein)
- ½ cup broccoli (2g protein)
- 2 tablespoons Salba seeds (2.6g protein)
- 1 cup cooked beans (16g protein)
- 1 cup cooked oat bran (7g protein)
- 1 plant-based protein smoothie (26g protein)
- 1 low-fat, no-sugar protein bar (10g protein)
- 50 grams almonds (11g protein)
- 100 grams pumpkin seeds (29g protein)
- 1 cup cooked pearled barley (5g protein)
- 1 avocado (4g protein)
- 1 baked potato, skin on (5g protein)
- 1 cup cooked lentils (18g protein)
- 1 cup cooked chickpeas (12g protein)

Vegetable-based proteins with all EAAs are the easiest to digest. Be sure to get the good proteins into your body and cut down on the bad ones.

The other side of the equation is the problem of eating too much protein. The average North American eats way more protein than is needed and consumes much more on average than those in any other developed country. Our BBQ-lovin' culture has resulted in a rich meat-based diet that has some not-so-great results. Anything in excess is a problem and too much unneeded protein in your body will be broken down and stored as fat. Diets that are very high in protein can also be hard on the body, potentially causing:

- High cholesterol levels due to lowered carbohydrate intake.
- Strain on your kidneys and liver, since unused protein must be broken down in the liver to separate out nitrogen waste which can lead to kidney stones.
- Excess uric acid in the bloodstream, which are toxic by-products of protein breakdown. This acid has to be pumped out by the kidneys which may result in the loss of essential minerals from the body including calcium. High uric acid is a preliminary factor in the development of gout and arthritis.
- Calcium-leeching from your bones, which weakens and may cause osteoporosis. (Note: a diet which contains 50 per cent more protein than is needed may result in as much as 1 per cent loss of bone mass a year.)

What exactly do you need?

The amount of protein you need each day depends on your age, level of exercise and gender. In general, it's recommended that 15-30 per cent of your daily calories come from protein: much less than most people eat. An easy way to determine the amount of protein you need is to take your body weight in pounds and divide by 22. Take this number and multiple by 0.8 if you are sedentary or 1.0-1.8 if you are very physically active, pregnant or under stress. This will give you the number of grams of protein that you need in a day.

Summary

Protein is an essential part of your body health. Ensuring you get all the EAAs in a day is an important aspect in providing your body with the essential building blocks it needs. Although animal food products contain all the EAAs, making them an easy choice, they have some negative aspects that should be considered before maxing out on them. Vegetable-based proteins are often not complete, but mixing and matching them can easily attain this. Conversely, opting for vegetable-based complete proteins like hemp, quinoa, buckwheat and amaranth are easy ways to ensure your whole protein needs get immediately met.

As North Americans we are blessed to have the problems that we do. Instead of the nutritionally-starved societies of other less-fortunate countries, on average we have too much protein in our daily diet food. By being aware of how much protein you really need and choosing sources that have few tag-alongs, you can make better choices that will deliver the biggest bang for your protein buck!

What you know now:
- Proteins, made up of EAAs, play a vital role in tissue development and are integral to your muscles, organs, bones and immune system.
- EAAs are just that: essential. They must be obtained through food sources.
- Pick your protein carefully to maximize the benefits it delivers; avoid proteins that have nasty tag-alongs.
- Know your limits and stick to them. Like anything in life, balance is the key. Too much protein is hard on your system and can have long term negative effects.

Apply to your daily routine:
- Eat a small amount of protein at every meal to spread it out throughout the day – dinner should not be your only source of protein!
- Jump-start your day with a plant-based protein smoothie or add a tablespoon of hemp seed to cereal each morning. For lunch, opt for a quinoa salad or green salad sprinkled with nuts. Do an easy

make-ahead vegetable-legume stew with barley, steel cut oats or buckwheat for dinner.

• Choose low-fat options of all animal-based proteins.

• Reduce or eliminate red meat and all processed meats, especially hot dogs and pepperoni pizza for children.

• Eat the protein you need and make sure you aren't on overdose mode.

• Get complete EAAs by mixing and matching for best results when eating plant-based options.

Conclusion

It's a very odd thing.
As odd as can be
That whatever Miss T. eats
Turns into Miss T.
Walter de la Mare, English poet and novelist (1873-1956)

Each pillar plays an important role in maintaining your health and well-being. When one is out of whack, your body has the intuitive ability to immediately respond in an attempt to always find balance. But your body is also your best friend who silently sends you signals as a plea for help. When you don't listen to it (for example, ignoring those aches and pains which are often the first signs of inflammation, or ignoring problems with your bowel movements, breathing and digestion), your body has no other option but to take matters into its own hands. When ignored, your body acts like a disgruntled lover who starts to tear apart the relationship due to a lack of attention.

The constant mode of trying to find a balance requires a lot of energy and work from your body. When you don't eat well, your body uses up energy in an attempt to find balance instead of using that energy in positive ways. This in turn causes your body stress. If this stress becomes chronic, eventually various parts of your system will become overworked and will begin to show signs of wear and tear. If left unchecked, it will manifest itself as an illness.

As a means of maintaining balance in the Temple of You, one of the easiest means is to consume foods that contain all three pillars. What kinds of foods are best for you? It's likely you've heard a great deal of media chatter about super foods, whole foods and maybe even raw foods. Let's look at these more closely.

Simply put, a whole food is one that has not been refined or processed. It is eaten in its natural state, such as fresh fruits and veggies. Whole foods may also include those that are cooked, such as rice or beans. A raw food is one that has not been heated above 118°F. This maintains all the natural enzymes and nutrients to aid in the digestive process. By default, a raw food is a whole food.

A whole food allows your body to work efficiently and to work less at processing the food, because all the nutrients are delivered immediately. Your body does not feel the need to hunt or sort for the various three pillars of nutrition, because you have delivered a complete package to its digestive door. What this means is that your body – being the wonderful construct that it is – can then focus its energy in other areas. It can fight off bacteria or viruses, rather than trying to figure out how to make sense of the poor foods you have fed it.

Simply put,
a whole food
is one that has
not been refined
or processed.

One of my friends, Brendan Brazier, is a competitive triathlete. He is in impeccable shape, trains hours a day and eats a mostly raw vegan diet. In his book, *The Thrive Diet*, he outlines his transition from a high-carb meat-based diet to a whole food, plant-based one. The result? He has become even more efficient – recovering faster and reducing stress and inflammation – by eating a 100 per cent plant-based diet. He says:

> "... as a general rule, the more processed the food is, the more stimulating its effect will be on the nervous system and the less nourishing. In contrast, the more natural and whole a food is—raw and sprouted being the best— the less stimulating and the more nourishing it will be."[14]

As a natural byproduct of a plant-based diet, your body becomes more pH balanced, because raw plant-based foods are alkaline in nature. Alkaline foods have minerals that leave an alkaline residue after food is consumed. Acidic foods leave an acidic residue. The pH scale goes from the most acidic rate of 1 to the most alkaline at 14. If too acidic, below the rate of 7.35, the body gets stressed, feels fatigued and has reduced immunity. Additionally, a long-term state of acidity can lead to kidney stones and a reduction of growth hormone levels which, means muscle loss and higher body fat as well as a loss of bone mass. Bacteria and viruses also love an acidic environment and cancer requires an acidic environment in which to live and grow.

So what are these acidic foods? Well, all these lovelies: animal proteins, white bread and white rice, cheese, sugar, alcohol, refined foods, caffeine, artificial sweeteners and tobacco. Alkaline foods include vegetables, beans, fresh fruits, maple syrup, lemons, plant-based protein, and chlorophyll-rich foods likeleafy greens. Just one more reason to order that salad!

I aspire to eat and work out like Brendan one day. Until then, I just try to be more like him and, hopefully, in 20 years I will be somewhere close to a 100 per cent plant-based diet and daily workouts. But, pending my retirement, I maintain a tight-wire act of trying to balance two young children, a hubby, a full-time job, two dogs, two horses, eight fish, one frog and a household of chaos and dirty dishes. But with a few changes, we can all become a little bit better.

Here are some principles to aim for:

- Eat at least one serving of raw foods or foods cooked at low temperature at each meal. This will get your digestion fired up and ready to pump through the processed or high-temperature-cooked foods faster.
- Choose whole, alkaline-forming foods to keep your body pH balanced. Start the day with a glass of lemon water to get alkalized first thing in the morning. Do a pH pee test each week to see where you are at – try to aim for 7.3. (You can find pH test strips at your drugstore or health food store.)
- Select natural and nutrient-rich foods to get your body working faster and more effectively.

By taking on these simple principles, you can reduce the amount of stress your body goes through when digesting processed or refined foods. The added bonus? You will need to eat less, because nutrient-rich foods keep your body nourished longer and turn off your brain's hunger signal. Most importantly, you are taking steps to reduce the risk of developing a number of diseases.

Now let's turn our attention to what some of the most common ailments are and what else you can actively do to prevent illness.

Three Major Threats to Better Being

. . . .

It seems, in fact, as though the second half of a man's life is made up of nothing but the habits he has accumulated during the first half.
Fyodor Dostoevsky, Russian author, (1821-1881)

Hopefully, you feel a little more comfortable in your knowledge of how your body works and are more aware of what you need to do to start repairing your lopsided Temple of You and make some better-for-you changes.

But the journey to better being also requires an understanding of some of the greatest risks to your health - risks exacerbated by not tending to your temple's pillars. The three greatest threats to North Americans' health are cardiovascular disease, cancer and diabetes. We will address each one of these to understand what they are, what causes them and what you can do to decrease your chances of getting them.

Heart Disease

Little privations are easily endured when the heart is
better treated than the body.
Jean Jacques Rousseau, Swiss philosopher (1712-1778)

During my teens I doubted my lofty legal aspirations once, when I had a nostalgic three-month period of one day becoming a veterinarian. I think this was during my "Buddhist phase," when I decided for a few months to trade in my family's Anglican virtues for the self-effacing Buddhist monk ones, much to my mother's horror.

However, my veterinary wistful dream was abruptly cut short when I got a job as an assistant in a vet clinic. The term "assistant" basically meant "whatever we, the vets, don't want to do, you get the pleasure of doing," so I did a lot of floor washing, bathing disgruntled dogs, cleaning out cages and initially assisting the doctors in surgery. The first few surgeries went relatively well as I successfully stopped myself from vomiting through deep breathing. However, the one that sent me over the precipice was a surgery being done on a cat. Let's just say that during this ordeal, I suddenly realized I could never be a vet and would gladly pay hefty vet bills for the rest of my animal-owning existence … then I passed out.

But what I saw that day has stayed with me all these years. It was the first and only time I saw a real heart. Let me just tell you that these throbbing suckers don't look at all like a Valentine's Day box of chocolates. Instead, it looks like a massive, diseased, rotting strawberry and to make matters worse, it pulsates. I still feel uncomfortable thinking about it. Surgery is definitely not my forte and I think the animal kingdom sleeps a little easier every night knowing I am not behind a knife. (By the way, the cat was fine and I never made it to the Buddhist monastery in Nepal.)

Although in reality it is not pretty to look at, this pulpy, pulsating powerhouse is truly amazing. As the second largest organ (the first being your skin) and your largest muscle, your heart is the life-sustaining motor that beats thousands of times each and every day to pump two thousand gallons of blood through your body! Sending blood around your body is a vital function, because blood contains oxygen, which is absorbed into your system through the lungs. This oxygen is then supplied to all your body's cells, which need the oxygen to live. Your heart also needs a steady supply of oxygen-rich blood to survive, so it pumps to feed itself, as well as to nourish the rest of the body.

But how does your heart work? Your heart is separated into a left and a right side with two chambers on each side that fill up with blood and then contract to squeeze the blood along to where it has to go. Each chamber has a door, or valve, that prevents the blood from escaping or flowing backwards. The top and bottom chambers work as a symbiotic tag team. The top chambers dump the returning blood into the bottom ones and then the bottom ones squeeze the blood out to the body and lungs. The act of moving the blood around your body is called circulation and amazingly, it takes just one minute for your heart to pump blood to every cell in your body, which is pretty impressive since there are trillions of them! So the better your circulation is, the faster your cells get fed.

As your cells use up the oxygen, they create carbon dioxide waste. This waste is taken away by the circulating blood and dumped into your lungs. As your blood is pumped into the lungs, the lungs take the carbon monoxide and discard it by sending it out in your exhaled breath. (Who knew your exhaled breath is really made up of cell garbage?) Then you inhale, fill up your system with oxygen and start feeding your cells once more. Your heart and the blood that pumps through your body basically act like a pizza delivery person who drives to your house, delivers the pizza and waits around to pick up the used paper pizza box, plates and cutlery and takes it all off to the recycling plant!

Heart health is key. Blocked heart arteries and the resulting heart attacks, are a leading killer in North America.

Cardiovascular Disease

Cardiovascular diseases (CVDs) are a group of disorders of the heart and blood vessels. Heart attacks and strokes are the most common CVDs and are mainly caused by a blockage of fatty deposits on the inner walls of the blood vessels.

This blockage prevents blood from flowing to the heart or the brain.

According to the World Health Organization, CVDs are on the increase worldwide and the numbers of those affected are staggering:[15]
- CVDs are the number one cause of death globally.
- In 2007, an estimated 17.1 million people died from CVDs, which represents 29 per cent of all global deaths. Of these deaths, an estimated 7.2 million were due to heart attacks and 5.7 million were due to strokes.
- By 2030, almost 23.6 million people will die from CVDs annually, mainly from heart disease and stroke.

Heart disease and strokes are projected to remain the single leading causes of death well into the future.

The World Health Organization states that unhealthy diet, physical inactivity and cigarette smoking is responsible for 80 per cent of all heart attacks.[16] How do you know if your poor choices make you a candidate for this disease? The effects of an unhealthy diet and physical inactivity often rear their ugly heads in ways such as high blood pressure, high blood sugar, raised blood fat levels and the obvious sign of being overweight or obese. These indicators become keystones for diagnosing higher risks of heart attack and stroke. Stress and old age can also add fuel to the CVD fire.

Unfortunately, there are often no symptoms of CVD and a heart attack or stroke may be the first warning of this underlying disease.

Symptoms of a heart attack include:
- Pain or discomfort in the centre of the chest
- Pain or discomfort in the arms, the left shoulder, elbows, jaw or back
- Shortness of breath
- Feeling sick or vomiting
- Feeling light-headed or faint
- Breaking into a cold sweat
- Becoming pale

I have had a couple of anxiety attacks at the worst times in my life and the symptoms were similar. One time, at the height of my 70-hour work weeks, I thought I was having heart failure at my desk. I tried to call 9-1-1 but couldn't because I could not identify the numbers on the touch pad. So even if you have had anxiety attacks in the past, don't discount these symptoms as "just stress" – whether you think it may be anxiety or not, you should get it checked out. And even if it is stress-related, you need to get that under control too, because your body is telling you that you need to chill out. (See "Mind Over Matter" section.)

Symptoms of a stroke include:
- Sudden weakness of the face, arm or leg (usually on one side of the body)
- Numbness of the face, arm or leg (usually on one side of the body)
- Disorientation
- Difficulty speaking or understanding speech
- Difficulty seeing
- Difficulty walking
- Loss of balance or dizziness
- Severe headache
- Fainting or unconsciousness

Basically, the symptoms of a stroke are what the average 20-year-old partygoer has at 3 a.m. on New Year's Day – but without any of the fun. There are a few things the average person can do to ensure they are not blindsided by these dangerous, but often silent, killers. The easiest is to have your blood pressure checked regularly. Basically, blood pressure measures how quickly and effectively your heart is pumping your blood around your body in its circulatory route. If your pressure is high, this means it takes more effort for your heart to push blood through your body and your blood takes longer to get where it needs to be. By measuring your blood pressure, you can see if there is any early warning sign of potential blockages.

What should you be aiming for? This following chart reflects blood pressure categories defined by the American Heart Association.

Blood Pressure Category	Systolic mm Hg (upper #)		Diastolic mm Hg (lower #)
Normal	less than 120	and	less than 80
Prehypertension	120 – 139	or	80 – 89
High Blood Pressure (Hypertension) Stage 1	140 – 159	or	90 – 99
High Blood Pressure (Hypertension) Stage 2	160 or higher	or	100 or higher
Hypertensive Crisis (Emergency care needed)	Higher than 180	or	Higher than 110

As high blood pressure has no symptoms, it is important to get your blood pressure checked regularly. Also opt for an annual blood sugar test and look out for the symptoms of high blood sugar levels, which can be a precursor to diabetes (more to come on this later). As diabetes greatly increases the risk of heart attacks and strokes, it is important to take active and easy steps to avoid developing diabetes. If you already have diabetes, make sure you vigilantly control your blood pressure and blood sugar to minimize your risk of CVD.

You now know that the heart is an amazing muscle and you need to keep it healthy. You also know that the biggest killer of North Americans is a silent sucker that lurks in fat-filled blood vessels. But what causes this blockage and what can you do to prevent this from happening?

Cholesterol

Talk about being misunderstood! Cholesterol, a kind of fat, probably gets the worst and most undeserved bad rap. Did you know that cholesterol is essential for all animal life and forms part of every cell in your body? It is also responsible for building the membranes in your cells, keeping your cells fluid, making some sex hormones and making vitamin D. This wax-like substance is found in animal fats (like meat, dairy, seafood and eggs) but is also naturally made in your liver. About 85 per cent of your blood cholesterol level is made by your body, with the remaining 15 per cent coming from your diet. It's a little goopy and can't move on its own, so it sticks to its best friend, protein, which then carries it around your blood highways.

There are two basic types of cholesterol, both of which are defined by how much protein is able to stick to it:

- Low-density lipoprotein (or LDL) cholesterol is low in protein, is very lethargic and is the EVIL cholesterol most likely to block up your blood vessels.
- High-density lipoprotein (or HDL) cholesterol has a lot of protein in it, acts efficiently and is the GREAT cholesterol that helps clear the LDL out of your blood and can reduce your risk for heart disease. HDL doesn't like the LDL too much – when it meets it, it grabs the LDL residue and dumps it in your liver to be sent out to the potty pasture.

Think of these two as competing twins: HDL is well-behaved and polite and LDL is the holy terror. There is no problem having a high level of HDL; in fact, it is something for which we all need to strive. The problem with cholesterol is not in having it, but in having too much of the bad kind.

Why is high LDL so bad? Simply put, having high LDL greatly increases your risk of coronary heart disease. Like a head cold that never ends, the stuffed up blood vessels prevent the blood from getting the necessary oxygen to your cells efficiently. So to protect your cells and make sure they don't die, your heart has to pump more blood and has to do it faster. The result? Your poor pulsating pump starts to wear out from fatigue and begins to weaken.

How do we get too much LDL? The average North American's love affair with TFA and S-Fat is a major dietary cause of high LDL levels. Like the bad relationship you stay in that you get nothing out of, it is time to just end it and send your bad fats walking.

Obesity

Being overweight or obese is also a risk factor to developing high LDL levels. Overweight and obese people on average have high LDL levels coupled with low HDL levels. This dangerous combo, along with other weight-driven effects, such as high blood pressure and inflammation, pose a major risk to your heart. Many medical symptoms common in overweight and obese people are also pre-diabetic, which is a big problem since developing diabetes significantly increases the risk of heart disease and higher mortality rates.

Smoking
Smoking is another cause of increased LDL. One of the 4,000 ingredients in cigarettes is something called acrolein. This substance is often used in pesticides to help kill insects and, if that weren't enough, it is often used in chemical weapons. Dee-lish. Once inhaled, acrolein is sent into your blood stream via your lungs. It changes the structure of LDL, which results in inflammation and plaque build-up. It also prevents HDL from carrying away fat, which increases your overall LDL cholesterol levels. The carbon monoxide in cigarettes also decreases the oxygen in your blood, which can lead to clots and clogged blood vessels. So if you needed yet another reason to quit, this has to rate as a good one!

Age & Gender
Age and gender can play a big role as well. LDL goes up after the age of 20 in both men and women and substantially increases after menopause for women. Women in this group should seriously look at their diet and ensure they prevent any LDL buildup before it happens. Men have a greater risk of having a heart attack (and earlier in life), but women are more likely to die from heart disease than from all the other major diseases combined (cancers, chronic lung disease, pneumonia, diabetes, accidents and AIDS).

Family Matters
Is there any good news? Absolutely! You now have something else to blame your parents for! Genes can also determine your propensity for having high LDL levels. These family jewels can play a role in making you more susceptible to diabetes, which can increase blood fat (triglycerides), which in turn can raise cholesterol levels. I highly recommend bringing up this tidbit of genetic blame over the next turkey and mashed spuds holiday meal. Your parents will thank me.

How much LDL is acceptable? The following is a general guideline for acceptable ranges:[17]

LDL Cholesterol Level	Classification
Less than 100 mg/dL	Desirable
100–129 mg/dL	Near optimal/above optimal
130–159 mg/dL	Borderline high
160–189 mg/dL	High risk
190 mg/dL and above	Very high risk

*If your total blood cholesterol level is greater than 200, test your LDL cholesterol, HDL cholesterol and triglycerides.

Total Cholesterol Level	Classification
Less than 200 mg/dL	Desirable
200–239 mg/dL*	Borderline high risk
240 mg/dL and above	Very high risk

HDL Cholesterol Level	Classification
Less than 40 mg/dL for men; less than 50 mg/dL for women	Major heart disease risk factor
60 mg/dL or higher	Gives some protection against heart disease

How can you prevent this sticky LDL goop floating around your body from sticking to something? The experts at Harvard Medical School reviewed this issue and found the answer is relatively simple. They came to the conclusion that a combination of different foods can help lower cholesterol by doing different but complimentary things. First, foods rich in S-Fibre (like beans, whole grains and oats) act as your body's buffed bouncer. S-Fibre grabs LDL cholesterol in your digestive system and drags it out before it gets too far. Second, eating P-Fats (like nuts and vegetable oils) can directly lower your LDL.

Researchers have also found regular exercise is a surefire way to reduce LDL. It has three benefits:

1. Reduces total blood cholesterol
2. Lowers LDL
3. Raises HDL

If you are exercising and losing weight, this also reduces your cholesterol risk. Being overweight can make your LDL cholesterol level go up and your HDL cholesterol levels go down ... so losing weight is a bonus fourth benefit of exercise!

Based on the very big brains at Harvard, here are some easy LDL balancing takeaways:

- Boost your daily consumption of fibre to 20 to 35 grams a day.
- Eat two ounces of nuts (1/2 cup) to reduce LDL by about five per cent.
- Eat a variety of S-Fibre and P-Fats to reduce the risk of high cholesterol.
- Start moving to raise your HDL and lower your LDL.

Additionally, other foods can assist in the LDL battle. Eat those veggies in raw form because recent research has found that veggies like broccoli strengthens and protects the heart due to its high levels of the phytochemical sulforaphane, which helps your body detoxify.[18] Other brassicus veggies like kale, cauliflower, cabbage, bok choy and Brussels sprouts will also do the trick. Adding garlic to your greens gets you an even bigger boost, as it has a complex array of phytochemicals that can help lower blood pressure and cholesterol levels.[19] Don't forget to keep your vitamin C levels up as well – this antioxidant protects the elastic strength of blood vessels and helps keep your circulation pristine.[20]

Increasing your gamma-linolenic acid (GLA) intake combined with omega-3 EFA's may help to reduce total LDL cholesterol and substantially reduce risks of heart attacks long term.[21]

Remember, small steps can have a huge impact: for every one per cent you lower your blood cholesterol level, you reduce your risk of heart disease by two per cent! Those are some not-so-Vegas "good" odds.

Summary

Your heart is the caregiver of your cells and works on overdrive when blood vessels are blocked. It is the motor upon which your life relies. When you don't take care of it, it just keeps on ticking until it cannot go any more. Heart disease is a huge killer, but because of few or no symptoms it can go undiagnosed until it is too late. Unfortunately, the risks of heart disease keep compounding, so each bad choice increases your risk. For example, if you have high LDL and you smoke and are overweight, then you are eight times more likely to develop heart disease than someone who has no risk factors.

By getting tested annually for blood pressure, blood sugar and cholesterol levels, you can educate yourself about your risk of harbouring this silent killer. Also, the great news is that you have the power to reduce these major risk factors and prevent cardiovascular disease through a healthy diet, regular physical activity and by quitting those cancer sticks!

What you know now:
- Your heart is your life pump that feeds oxygen to each one of your cells while also helping discard waste through your blood vessel highways.
- Blockages in your blood vessels filled with LDLs can lead to the silent killers: strokes and heart attacks.
- Reduce the risk of developing blocked arteries rich in LDL by: (1) make healthy food choices, (2) quit smoking, (3) exercise and (4) maintain a healthy weight.

Apply to your daily routine:
- Have five servings of fruits and vegetables a day to help raise your HDL levels.
- Get your daily fibre fix with 20-35 grams per day.
- Choose a P-Fat (EFAs please!) over any other for an added HDL boost. Combine with GLA rich-foods for added protection.
- Be active daily – opt for a 10-minute walk instead of a 10-minute cigarette break.
- Just say NO to ciggies … and wait for your 80th birthday to start again with the rest of us addicts (more on this later!).
- Get an annual test to check blood pressure, blood sugar and cholesterol levels.

Cancer

It isn't what we don't know that gives us trouble;
it's what we know that ain't so.
Will Rogers, cowboy and comedian (1879-1935)

I have only physically assaulted a doctor on one occasion and luckily my sister was there to drag me off him. It happened in the palliative care section of the hospital where my mother was being "cared" for. She fought lung and breast cancer for over a year and was losing the war. Her body had become the zone in which all battles took place.

After nursing her at home for more than a year, mostly by my sister and father, our family succumbed to the harsh reality that she needed to be in a hospital and would likely not return home. My family did hospital shifts so she was never alone. We also took her our own home-cooked meals, as a fast review of the meal trays revealed that the hospital meals were all cancer-inducing pots of schlop. At this stage, though, she was eating so little it did not really matter.

I was due to start my shift on a Sunday morning at two a.m. I went into the hospital pumped up from the four hours of dancing I had just done at a dance club, trying to lose myself in the music and prevent any thoughts from entering my brain. As I entered the hospital ward I heard blood-curdling screams and I knew it was her.

A lot of cancers cause a great deal of pain when they develop and spread. In palliative cases, doctors usually prescribe massive amounts of pain medication, like morphine, to make it easier on the patient. In this case, her administering doctor had not written on her chart that she could have painkillers and the on-call emergency doctor decided that he wouldn't give it to her until he could speak with her treating doctor. Her treating doctor was, not surprisingly, unavailable at 2 a.m. on a Sunday morning. So after yelling expletives at him, I made a flying leap towards him in a desperate act to pin his body against the hallway wall. Now, I would not recommend this behaviour to anyone, as first of all, it is illegal (assault) and second of all, it can really harm someone. But at the young age of 21, pumped up on dance tunes combined with an all encompassing desire to get my mom pain relief, it seemed like a viable option. Since I was at the height of my eating disorder and weighed an intimidating 102 pounds, I was not really a threat to anything other than a small animal. My sister maturely intervened and plucked me off the embarrassed man. After a negotiation that felt like an eternity, he finally agreed to administer the sleepy-time drugs my mother needed. She died four days later in my and my sister's arms. She was only 56 years old.

As I sit here writing this, some 20 years later, the sadness of this loss has not subsided and tears still roll down my face. But from any experience comes the potential to learn and trust me when I say that I had a lifetime of lessons that came out of this one! But now my goal is to make sure I live as long as I can and have the experience of watching my children grow to their greatest potential and, hopefully, to be so blessed as to meet and greet my future grandkids. The quest for health is all about buying time and having as much of it as possible on our wonderful planet. Let's figure out what you can do to help reduce your risks and remain cancer-free.

So what is this infamous disease?

Cancer is a group of many related diseases that all share one thing in common: deviant cell growth. Starting out normal, a cell becomes damaged for a number of reasons, both naturally and as a result of external factors. The damaged cell then genetically mutates over time to become a cancer cell. These changes can happen naturally, like when a cell divides it may inadvertently cause damage to itself. You can also be born with a genetic mutation that makes you more susceptible to a particular kind of cancer passed down through your genes. But there are also known causes of cell damage that are caused by human-made carcinogens.

Instead of a normal cell that knows when to grow, when to stop growing and when to die, abnormal cancer cells continue to grow and just don't know when to stop. Like Arnold Schwarzenegger in the *Terminator*, they just keep going and going. They are birds of a feather and like to clump together, making tumors which proceed to destroy the normal cells around them. They love to vacation in exotic places and travel around to other areas, quickly spreading out. There are lots of cancers to pick from with over 200 different kinds!

Cancer symptoms are quite varied and depend on the type of cancer and whether it has spread. Typically, early symptoms include fatigue, fever, weight loss, anemia and sweating because the growth of any cancer uses up the body's energy.

Treatment is diverse, also depending on the type of cancer and how much it has spread. Most common treatments include surgical removal, chemotherapy (ingested drugs) and radiation (high energy waves). All of these traditional cancer treatments can damage healthy cells in the process of trying to get rid of the cancerous ones, with chemotherapy being the most extreme. It is a bit like Russian roulette in that what is targeted is inexact. There are other non-traditional less invasive approaches such as naturopathic treatments that may be taken in conjunction with traditional medicine or as a stand-alone approach.

Although experts do not know exactly what causes cancer, they do know that damaged cells have a greater risk of developing it. When exposed to carcinogens (such as tobacco, exhaust fumes, x-rays, sun rays, radiation and asbestos) or when cells become damaged naturally or by a genetic predisposition, your body creates highly reactive molecules known as free radicals. Free radicals are directly responsible for damaging a cell's DNA and for promoting a cancer-loving environment. Free radicals are damaged molecules missing an electron so they hunt around your body looking to steal electrons from other healthy molecules. Like crazed bumper cars, they knock into other molecules within your cells looking to steal an electron, which can result in damage to your proteins, membranes and genes.

This free radical damage, researchers believe, is likely the cause of cancer and Alzheimer's and speeds up the body's aging process. Additionally, once the free radical steals an electron from another molecule, that molecule in turn becomes damaged. When the first mutant cell divides, the molecule mutation is passed on to other cells and so on and so on and so on. These mutated cells are receptive to cancer because their strength is reduced from the mutation. So the more free radicals you have in your body, the higher your risk of getting cancer.

There is no single cause for any one type of cancer and there is little known about why cancer is so prevalent. Even though the cause (and cure) is undiscovered, researches do know there are certain contributors to increased cancer risk.

Immunity

Low immune systems and aging bodies are both prime targets for cancer, as these normal cells are more susceptible to outside forces. By boosting your immune system and reducing symptoms of aging by staying healthy, you can decrease your risk levels. There are many foods that can assist in strengthening the immune system. Chlorella can remove toxic metals that exacerbate free radical activity. Foods rich in antioxidants (like vitamin C, selenium and carotenoids) can assist in cell-protection and regeneration and also mop up the free radicals. These foods include citrus fruits, strawberries, broccoli, green peppers, carrots, kale, sweet potatoes, squash, thyme and cilantro. Antioxidant-rich vitamin E foods produce immune cells that destroy bacteria and include grains, seeds and vegetable oils. EFA omega-3-rich foods can also increase the bustle of bacteria-eating cells. Infection-fighting zinc is found in seeds, chickpeas and lentils and garlic has incredible immunity attributes.

Obesity

Researchers know that being overweight increases your risk of bowel cancer and pancreatic cancer. Obesity and inactivity can also increase your risk of esophageal cancer, kidney cancer, gallbladder cancer and, in women, breast or uterine (womb) cancer.[22] Try to maintain your weight at a healthy, stable level. If you are obese or overweight, now is a good time to get motivated to get rid of some pounds.

Alcohol

Sorry to be the bearer of bad news, but drinking alcohol has been found to increase the risk of liver cancer, bowel cancer and, most dramatically, breast cancer. I know ... heavy sigh inserted here! Research done on more than a million British women identified that for every extra daily unit of alcohol (over two a week), the risk for breast cancer increases by one per cent.[23] So teetotalers unite and take over!

Sun

Fun in the sun – or too much of it – greatly increases the risk of skin cancer. Get your 15 minutes of sun for your vitamin D boost, but after that cover up and enjoy the shade! Remember, ultraviolet (UV) radiation comes from the sun, sunlamps and tanning booths, so be aware of the damage from tans. Although it may look good, a tan is a sign you have damaged your biggest organ: the skin. Do a skin check monthly and watch for any moles that change shape or colour.

Smoking

Tobacco is downright evil. Smokers are more likely than nonsmokers to develop cancer of the lung, voice box, mouth, throat, stomach, pancreas, esophagus, bladder, kidney, cervix and blood (leukemia).[24] But the good news is that the risk of cancer for people who quit is lower than the risk for people who continue to use tobacco. The risk of cancer is lowest among those who never used tobacco so if you are thinking of starting … just DON'T. If you are a smoker, take the plunge and quit now. Send that cancer risk up in smoke!

BBQing

Speaking of smoke, smoking and barbecuing meat produces two types of potentially carcinogenic compounds: polycyclic aromatic hydrocarbons (PAHs) found mainly in smoked foods and heterocyclic amines (HCAs) found mainly in charred food. Both are suspected of causing cancer in humans.[25] Here are some simple steps to reduce your risks: (1) minimize eating bar-b-qued, grilled and smoked food, (2) use meats that have a lower fat content and remove excess fat, (3) turn down the high heat and opt for a medium or low heat slow cook, (4) remove charred areas before eating and (5) marinate![26]

Chemicals

People who are exposed to radiation or who work with environmental contaminants such as paint, pesticides, chemicals or construction materials have an increased risk of cancer. Many studies have shown that exposure to asbestos, benzene, benzidine, cadmium, nickel or vinyl chloride in the workplace can cause cancer.[27] Exposure to diesel exhaust fumes over long periods of time also increases your risk of lung cancer.[28] Stay away from these substances as best you can and only have x-rays when medically necessary.

Acidity

Last but not least, your pH balance is vital to your body health. Advertisiers tell us that pH balance is an issue for healthy hair, but it's more of a whole body concern. Your body tries constantly to balance its pH levels. When the levels are too acidic, it affects your health at a cellular level as inflammation is bred and viruses and bacteria thrive. When alkaline (meaning balanced), cancer cannot survive and inflammation is kept to a minimum. Processed and refined foods that are denatured are acid-forming and create toxins in your body, yet they hold their high caloric amounts. What a horrible combination! Additionally, most synthetic vitamins, artificial sweeteners and prescription drugs are acid-forming. There are many pH-balanced foods, most of which are raw, unprocessed and whole foods. These include bananas, figs, citrus fruits (acidic at first but metabolized as alkaline), hemp seeds, and all vegetables that are green in colour (i.e. rich in chlorophyll).

Although no foods have been proven to combat ALL cancers, researchers do know that fruits, vegetables, seeds and nuts can protect against cancers of the upper digestive system, such as the mouth, esophagus and stomach. While fruits and veggies won't cure a cancer, researchers are fairly sure folate and vitamins A and C play an important role in protecting against it.[29] Broccoli and broccoli sprouts can help reduce the risks of cancer of the stomach, pancreas, lung, breast, prostrate, oveary and colon.[30] A diet high in carotenoids (the antioxidant pigments that give whole foods their colour) can help reduce ovarian cancer risks.[31] Gamma-linolenic acid has been found to increase the effectiveness of drugs used to treat breast cancer[32] and can inhibit the cancer gene responsible for over 30 per cent of all breast cancers.[33] Fibre, not surprisingly, can assist in reducing bowel cancer. One study showed that people who ate the most fibre had a 40 per cent lower risk of bowel cancer than those who ate the least.[34] Some studies have linked red and processed meat to cancer of the colon, prostrate, breast, bladder and stomach, so lay off the steak (and the barbeque)!

But whatever you do, remember that food is your best source of vitamin and minerals as supplements just don't cut it. Some research even suggests they can do more harm than good.[35] Also remember that cooking does diminish the nutrients in fruits, nuts, seeds and vegetables, so eat them in their beautiful raw form as often as you can.

When you choose to get your nutrients in the instant delivery system Mother Nature intended by eating raw whole foods, you can instantly accomplish several things: you receive the natural enzymes in raw form that promote a healthier gut and allow for better digestion; you receive micronutrients (vitamins and minerals) your body needs and craves; and, you alleviate stress on your system because your body intuitively knows how to process these foods, avoiding the heroin-type reaction that occurs when you consume processed foods.

Summary

The scary thing about cancer is you don't know you have it until it has manifested itself and taken hold on some level. Because it is internal and unseen, with few clear symptoms, it cannot be easily diagnosed in its infancy stage. Although researchers do not know the clear cause nor do they have a cure for it, they do know this illness happens over time. As such, it is important to take preventative steps early on in order to ensure this mutant monster is kept at bay. The easiest way to do so is to ensure free radicals are decreased and risk factors are kept to a minimum.

Although increased risk factors include situations often not in your control, there are major risk factors that can be controlled. By conscientiously reducing your risks with a couple of simple tweaks to your lifestyle you can get going down a cancer-free path.

What you know now:

- Cancer happens over time and includes a number of diseases that attack certain areas of your body through deviant cell growth.
- There is no known cause or cure, but research suggests there are known risks, both natural and human-made, that elevate your chances of getting cancer.
- To reduce major risks that are within your control:

- Keep your immune system strong
- Maintain a healthy weight
- Exercise
- Lay off the booze
- Stay in the shade
- Quit the ciggies
- Barbeque in a smart way
- Stay away from known carcinogenic toxins
- Take a pH balance test weekly with over-the-counter alkalinity swabs
- Eating antioxidant-rich raw fruit and veggies along with seeds, nuts and fibre rich foods will help to pump up your immune system, decrease free radicals and keep your body strong.

Apply to your daily routine:

- Limit exposure to man-made chemical carcinogens. Use toxic-free paint and cleaning products in your home.
- Make small changes that add up over time. Opt to walk or take public transit instead of taking the car and in order to reduce exposure to fumes, never allow your car to idle.
- Boost your immune system daily with simple additions like chlorophyll rich foods and add antioxidant-rich free-radical-preventing foods like berries, nuts and seeds to your snacks and breakfast.
- Get alkaline each morning by drinking a glass of water with a lemon wedge squeezed in. Become pH-balanced before you even walk out the door!
- Before reaching for that alcohol-infused cocktail, opt for a green tea that is calorie free and has antioxidants, which may slow down cancer growth.
- Shake your thing and move it to reduce it.
- Put your ciggies to rest – or else they may be doing it to you (permanently)!

Diabetes

The body never lies.
Martha Graham, dancer and choreographer (1894-1991)

I lived as a diabetic virgin until the ripe old age of 20. That was when I met my friend Jay. He was a guy I went to university with who became my study partner. He told me he was diabetic and it had the same impact as if he had told me he lived on the planet Zinglon, as I had never been exposed to diabetes. His illness did not sink in until the day he came to my house to study for an exam and he gave himself a needle. Being needle-phobic, I was horrified to watch him nonchalantly bring it out and stick it in his arm. I had no idea that people had to administer their own needles on a daily basis – what a horrible existence, I thought! He was great about educating those around him about his illness and I learned a lot. But he was the only one I knew who had diabetes up until my mid 30s.

Fast forward to the present and it is incredible how many people I meet at shows and events who are diabetic or pre-diabetic. Why this sudden influx? The number of people with type 2 diabetics has drastically increased in the last two decades. The Centers for Disease Control now recognize it as an epidemic based upon the rate it has increased and the number of people it now affects. It is one of the fastest-growing diseases in Canada, with over 60,000 new cases reported per year. A shocking total of 1.3 million Canadians and 24 million Americans are currently diagnosed with type 2 diabetes with future expected rates to exponentially increase. The crazy thing is, this disease is largely preventable through simple changes to diet and levels of exercise.

As you now know, whenever you eat food, the sugar in it (glucose) is absorbed from your intestines and distributed by the bloodstream to all the cells in your body. If anything is left over, your body stores the excess in the liver and muscles by creating long chains of glucose. When your body needs food (glucose) your pancreas secretes a hormone called glucagon, which results in your body sourcing and releasing the stored glucose and lets you know it is time to eat. Conversely, when you do eat and too much glucose is in your system, your pancreas secrets insulin in order to decrease blood sugar levels by assisting the transportation of glucose into the body's cells and to stop the secretion of glucagon, which triggers the release of stored glucose into the blood. To maintain a constant blood-glucose level, your body relies on your pancreas to act as your body's sugar teeter-totter and intuitively know when to secret the insulin and the glucagon. (See "The Three Pillars" for a reminder of the working of the pancreas.)

Diabetes is classified into three types: type 1, type 2 and gestational diabetes.

Type 1 Diabetes

Juvenile diabetes or insulin-dependent diabetes, usually diagnosed in childhood, results from a lack of insulin production by the pancreas and represents about 5-10 per cent of diabetics. In type 1 diabetics, the pancreatic areas that produce insulin are actually destroyed by the person's own immune system, genetics or environmental factors. This type requires injections of insulin daily and glucose levels need to be reviewed many times throughout the day. As well, those with type 1 diabetes need to keep a close watch on carbs and fat foods in their diet.

Type 2 Diabetes

Adult-onset diabetes or non-insulin-dependent diabetes occurs when the body is insulin resistant. The body can't use its own insulin, which means there are higher-than-normal levels of insulin in the blood. Depending on the severity of the diabetes, oral medication may be required and blood glucose levels should be reviewed. This type represents 90-95 per cent of diabetics and usually occurs in adults over the age of 40, although the number of adolescent diabetes is increasing at an alarming rate. With more than 180,000 Canadian children with this disease, Canada has the sixth highest incidence rate for children 14 years or younger in the world.

What happened to make a preventable disease such an epidemic? *Lack of exercise, inflammation due to a high fat diet and nutrient lacking insulin-spiking food consumption is the major cause of this dramatic increase.* Research has also linked type 2 risks with obesity, so the more overweight you are, the more likely you are to get this disease in the future.

Gestational Diabetes

Gestational diabetes can occur in some pregnant women and is similar to type 2 diabetes. It is believed gestational diabetes is caused by the hormones produced during pregnancy which likely increase a woman's resistance to insulin, with the result of impaired glucose tolerance. This type of diabetes usually goes away after delivery, but having it does increase your chances of developing type 2 diabetes later in life.

Diabetes is an incurable disease that affects your body's ability to use glucose. All diabetic symptoms include:

- Unexplained weight loss
- Excessive thirst
- Frequent urination
- Extreme hunger
- Numbness or tingling in hands and feet
- Slow-healing sores
- Unexplained high frequency of infection
- Glucose in the urine
- Unexplained fatigue
- Poor vision

What happens when you have no insulin or insulin resistance? It basically causes a reduced sugar (glucose) tolerance, as your cells cannot absorb glucose from your bloodstream. As a result, your blood-glucose levels rise when you are not eating, or after a meal. With no glucose coming from your blood, your body is tricked into thinking you are starving it. To respond, your pancreas tries to rebalance itself by secreting glucagon, which acts on your liver, kidneys and muscles to release more glucose, thereby raising your blood-glucose levels even more.

A lack of insulin or insulin-resistance and the ensuing high blood sugar (glucose) levels have incredibly damaging effects and can result in:

- Kidney stress because the kidneys have to work in overdrive mode to filter out all the increased glucose roaming around.
- Fatty acid metabolization, which leads to the production of acidic ketones in the blood and can cause breathing problems, heart irregularities and central-nervous system depression.

- Starved cells with nothing to burn for energy, as they cannot absorb glucose.
- High blood glucose levels, which cause poor blood circulation and increase the osmotic pressure of your blood. This increased pressure dehydrates your tissues, as water is drawn from your cells.
- Kidneys disposing of the water in your blood, as urine – which results in blood volume – decreases, causing thickening of the blood and poor circulation so your heart has to work so much harder to do the same job.

Additionally, cardiovascular disease (CVD) is a major complication of diabetes and is the leading cause of early death among people with diabetes.

- About 65 per cent of people with diabetes die from heart disease and stroke.[36]
- Adults with diabetes are two to four times more likely to have heart disease or suffer a stroke than people without diabetes.[37]
- High blood glucose in adults with diabetes increases the risk for heart attack, stroke, angina and coronary artery disease.[38]
- People with type 2 diabetes also have high rates of high blood pressure, lipid problems and obesity, which contribute to their high rates of CVD.[39]
- Smoking doubles the risk of CVD in people with diabetes.[40]

What can be done?

Balanced Diet

Because food affects blood sugar levels, ensuring you get a healthy and balanced diet is key to the prevention and treatment of diabetes. To assist in blood sugar metabolization eat foods rich in chromium (whole grains), manganese (brown rice, chickpeas and almonds), silicon (strawberries, leeks and spinach) and zinc (nuts, dry beans and pumpkin seeds). Cinnamon can improve insulin resistance and ginger can improve blood sugar control, so keep these great-tasting spices front and centre in your cooking. Diabetics are victims of low magnesium, which can worsen the complications of diabetes, especially type 2. Magnesium helps to metabolize glucose, so reach for the leafy greens, beans, whole grains, nuts and seeds.

Soluble Fibre

S-Fibre can slow down digestion and the speed at which carbs are absorbed in the intestines. Foods such as kidney beans, lentils and chickpeas are great options. Salba is a simple solution and can be sprinkled on salads, oatmeal and yogurt and in smoothies. According to peer-reviewed research on type 2 diabetics, daily doses of Salba (Salvia hispanica L) has the ability to reduce:

- After-meal blood sugar levels resulting in less insulin spikes.
- Blood pressure, which is the major cardiovascular risk factor in type 2 diabetics.
- Blood clotting by 21 per cent (without affecting coagulation).
- Inflammation levels by 40 per cent (C-Reactive Proteins).[41]

This easy and tasteless high-fibre addition is a no-brainer.

Reduce Processed Foods

Stay away from the inflammatory and empty calories, found in white flour and refined foods. S-Fat- and TFA is commonly found in processed foods and creates stress on the pancreas and liver, so reduce and/or eliminate these bad fats to ensure your pancreas works more efficiently.

Cut Sugar

Obviously, a reduction in sugar is required, so opt for non-spiking agave nectar (from a cactus plant), which is sinfully sweet with a low insulin response and does not have the blood glucose spikes caused by refined sugar. Also, cut out the fruit juices unless freshly squeezed to ensure you reap the benefits of the fibre and enzymes. Don't drink soda pop – EVER! The sugary kind is diabetes in a can and the artificially sweetened ones are potential carcinogens. If you need to get in your daily bubbles, opt for sparkling water with a twist of lemon.

Eat Regularly

Graze rather than eating large portions as this is less stressful on your body and allows for more efficient digestion. Remember: keep portions small!

Get Active
Stay active! Exercise assists in lowering blood sugar levels.

Quit Smoking
Okay, okay, I will say this one more time: QUIT SMOKING. (Yes, now I'm yelling.) This really is getting silly if you are still at it.

Summary
Diabetes is a damaging disease that has destructive effects on major organs in your system. Although gestational and type 1 diabetes cannot be prevented, their effects can be very well managed with changes to diet and exercise. So watch what you eat and get up and go!

Type 2 diabetes is commonly preventable and can be managed with a nutrient rich diet and by adopting an active lifestyle. The answers to this one are clearly that simple. Enough said!

What you know now:
- Diabetes is at epidemic levels and is a disease which can have very damaging effects upon the kidneys. It predisposes you to heart disease comes in three forms – one of which is entirely preventable based upon good lifestyle choices.
- The negative effects of diabetes can be substantially reduced by making better food choices that lower blood sugar levels and by remaining physically active.

Apply to your daily routine:
- Use the medically-studied Salba (Salvia hispanica L) daily to reduce effects of diabetes and its inherent CVD risks.
- Be active, not reactive. Get exercising to reduce risks rather than wait for it to happen once you have let yourself go too far. If you already have diabetes, reduce the damage that can be done by getting the exercise you need to reduce blood sugar levels.
- Eat foods daily that are fibre-rich and green and leafy and get your beans, nuts and seeds in.
- Quit smoking! (Sounding like a broken record here.)

Conclusion

Everything that used to be a sin is now a disease.

Bill Maher, American comedian, actor, writer and producer (b. 1956)

So you now know what can happen if your Temple becomes lopsided for long periods of time. Like a garden that is left to fend for itself, when you leave your body unattended the weeds need to be plucked and cleared before any new healthy growth can occur. The weeds in the case of the body are pretty simple and there are very clear steps that are required when you want to decrease your overall risks.

I think that the World Health Organization lays it out best in the following chart No more explaining required!

Risk Factor	Cardiovascular Diseases*	Diabetes	Cancer
Smoking	√	√	√
Alcohol	√		√
Physical Inactivity	√	√	√
Nutrition	√	√	√
Obesity	√	√	√
Raised Blood Pressure	√	√	
Dietary Fat/Blood Lipids	√	√	√
Blood Glucose	√	√	√

*This included heart disease, stroke and hypertension.

Source: World Health Organization

Mind Over Matter

. . . .

Be who you are and say what you feel because those
who mind don't matter and those who matter don't mind.
Dr. Seuss, children's author and amazing person (1904-1991)

In addition to understanding your body, it is also imperative for overall well-being to understand your mind. The two work in tandem and both have to be balanced. No matter how much good food and exercise you get, if you are out of whack upstairs, it will manifest itself physically elsewhere.

I found it a strange dichotomy that a particularly expensive health food store in a chi-chi area close to my old workplace had the rudest and most miserable staff. After studying them closely I realized they were wretched because the well-heeled customers treated them with distain and arrogance. Let's be clear on this: health and well-being does not depend upon a "holier than thou" mentality or living in a high-income neighborhood in a big city centre.

You can have the most expensive designer handbag in the world and eat organic food out the ying-yang, but this will not change the damage being done on the inside if you have negative thoughts and a judgmental attitude. Conversely, someone can have little financial means, but make good daily choices and have an excellent outlook on life, which will result in health and happiness.

Let's look at some of the key points to look out for from a mental standpoint and how you can work around these pitfalls to allow you to build the better you.

The Dangers of Diets

I've been on a constant diet for the last two decades. I've lost a total of 789 pounds. By all accounts, I should be hanging from a charm bracelet.
Erma Bombeck, American humorist (1927-1996)

During my early 30's, with a marriage breaking up, a 70-hour a week job and desperately trying to climb up the lame corporate ladder of life, I decided right before a business trip to shed a few extra pounds. I embarked upon a "cleanse" that required me to reduce consumption of most foods and to take some pills along with a horrible concoction a few times a day. I have since learned that just as "muffin" is another word for "cake," "cleanse" is another word for "diet."

While on the plane heading to the southern states, I felt the first sense of queasiness that soon turned into full-on flu-like systems. Now I don't know about you, but there is truly no way to hide much that is happening from those around you while packed into a tin can in the sky. What was worse was that I was travelling with my then-senior executive boss. I spent a good part of the journey locked in the restroom feeling sick, embarrassed and highly claustrophobic. It also didn't help that I am a germaphobe, so every visualization of the myriad of bacteria lurking in that small trunk of a restroom just perpetuated my nausea.

Lucky for me, once we landed we had a four-hour drive ahead of us. Let me tell you – for career growth, there is truly nothing as advancing as throwing up by the side of an interstate highway, while your boss waits for you in a rental car. I thought fast on my woozy feet and blamed it on "female issues," since no man can have any reasonable response to this statement.

Needless to say, I immediately stopped the cleanse and ordered up some Pepto when I finally got to the hotel. Looking back, I honestly see what a truly ridiculous decision it was to embark on a new diet in order to try to be the human lollipop that I aspired to resemble.

But you know, we have all done it. Think of that fateful morning when you step out of bed and realize that you feel lethargic and bloated. While showering, you look down at your stomach and thighs and think some alien infiltrated your body overnight and expanded your skin. While reviewing yourself in the mirror (face only) you mentally articulate your devastating realization: "Wow, I feel so … so fat." In a desperate measure to convince yourself otherwise, you try to ram your behind into the pants that are usually just a "little snug." This time, unfortunately, they are not just snug but are simply unwearable, like everything else in your closet. "Ugh," you think, "yet another expensive shopping trip to buy a pair of 'big pants'."

What happens next is the mental mind game that is debilitating: low self-esteem and feelings of inadequacy quickly set in. Slender people become the focus of your wrath, as you glare at them while telling yourself they must just have good genes and they have it so easy. Then the fateful day comes when you embark upon that life-changing moment: you decide to diet.

With best intentions, you take on the challenge to shed your skin, convincing yourself that it is possible to lose ten pounds in ten days – the before and after testimonials on the television prove it! You can become your former 16-year-old svelte self. This time you can complete the diet, because the "short-term pain will result in long-term gain."

Once you have decided upon your impending metamorphosis, a start date is chosen, which is usually on a Monday. This projected beginning allows you to have one last celebration with the food and drink you will be denied in your new regimen. Woo-hoo! When you have to lose 20 pounds, what's another two to lose after a "good" binge weekend?

You start the new program with vigor and drive … until around the third day. Your good intentions slowly begin to crumble as your body starts to crave what it knows so well: bad fats, sugar, starch and fried foods. You haven't eaten chocolate mousse for six months but by day three you are craving that creamy fat-laden treat and dream of being dipped in a vat of it.

By day four, you now know it is no accident that the word's first three letters spell D-I-E, as once you are into it you feel like life as you know it has ended forever. Your stomach is turning itself inside out due to gurgling and the sweats and cramping are overwhelming … you've had the flu with less severe symptoms! How can anyone sustain themselves on such a minimal amount of food?

By day five your wrath is focused upon the diet's creators. How could they have been so cruel and mean to devise such torture-laden plans? Rabbits eat more than this! Every thought you have is about food and what you could be eating at this very moment, if not for this four letter word: D-I-E-T.

By day seven the little voices in your head have started talking back:
• "Just one little 'snack' won't make a difference."
• "It is not 'cheating' if it is a special event."
• "I lost a couple of pounds so a little reward for a job well done won't hurt."

Even if you are able to stay focused and remain on the diet, once it has ended, it is not long before you fall back into your old habits and the cycle eventually starts all over again.

If this sounds like you, just find comfort in knowing you are not alone in this pattern of behavior. In fact, approximately 46 per cent of North American men and women initiate weight loss in any given year and 84 per cent use a change in diet to get results.[42] It is not surprising, given we are bombarded with visuals of Hollywood starlets who are shockingly underweight. Little do we know that these quaffed skeletons employ full time personal trainers, wardrobe consultants, graphic artists (to airbrush away their nutritionally deprived pimply skin), hairstylists and makeup artists to assist them in their unattainable looks. If Marilyn Monroe auditioned for a leading lady role in today's world she would be told to take some diet pills and come back when she was 20 pounds lighter!

Other than the psychological damage diets force upon you, what is most disconcerting about this North American phenomenon is the fact that it doesn't work. Let me say this one more time: IT DOES NOT WORK. If it did, the weight management industry, with revenues of approximately

$55 BILLION, would be out of business![43] Not only does it statistically not help to shed the pounds, but yo-yo dieting has the added effect of steady weight gain.

A recent medical study reviewed the long-term outcome of calorie-restricting diets. The outcome? One-third to two-thirds of dieters regained more weight over time than they initially lost on their diets. Additionally, there was no consistent evidence that dieting results in any kind of significant health improvement, no matter how much weight is lost. In fact, there is little evidence that diets lead to any lasting weight loss or health benefits.[44]

Why is this the case?

Your body is made up of 70 per cent water. So when you get the flu for 48 hours and think the only benefit is that you became slimmer, it is because you are dehydrated and have lost water not fat. You are in effect a human pickle. Likewise, to get fast results, many commercial diets are based on dehydration techniques to make it easier to lose the 10 pounds of water within several days.

Your body is smart. When you suddenly give it fewer calories it starts to adjust and says, "Hmm ... I'd better save some for later, as I don't know what this lunatic is going to do next!" So your body slows your metabolism down to adjust to the reduced intake. But listen up here – a diet without an increase in exercise will result in a reduction in lean muscle mass before fat will be reduced. It is estimated that when you lose two pounds or more per week, 30-40 per cent of the weight loss is actually muscle.

With muscle being five times more "active" than fat (meaning by just being there muscle burns off five times more calories than the fat that is sitting around), when you deplete your muscle mass it becomes even harder to keep the weight off in the long term. It becomes a crazy cycle, because the reduction of muscle causes an even greater reduction in your metabolism. With a lowered metabolism, you need to eat even fewer calories to lose any weight. Also, by dieting alone, if you stop your diet or go back to old eating habits, the weight will come back on even faster because your body, with less muscle, is burning far fewer calories per day. Even worse is that weight gain after a diet is mostly fat rather than the muscle you lost.

You now know that being overweight or obese is a serious health risk, not to mention a self-esteem breaker. So if dieting doesn't work, what can be done?

The best thing you can start doing is to take baby steps. By reducing calories gradually over time you will readjust your metabolism with long-term effects (say 100 calories a week for one month, then an additional 100 calories the second month and so on). By doing so, you can make a long-term difference. These changes can be simple ones that are easy to adhere to, such as opting for milk instead of cream in coffee or having fruit instead of cookies for a snack each day. Over time, instead of gaining a few pounds each year (which over ten years results in the panic diet mode) you can shed a few each year with long-term benefits and results. Your metabolism will gradually adjust, allowing for maintenance of your muscle mass and allowing your body to burn the fat off.

Feed your body with energy-rich foods, not empty calories high in fat and salt. By incorporating good foods you will start to see and feel a difference. Try a protein-rich smoothie every morning to kick start your day, or an energy-dense bar for a snack that gets you to dinner without overeating when you sit down. The low energy mood swings of the past will give way to feelings of empowerment and oomph!

Another thing you have to do is MOVE. I am not going to lecture you about the 30 x 4 rule (30 minutes of aerobic activity like a brisk walk, running, biking or swimming for 4 times a week) as a core part of remaining fit. This is what we all aspire to do but end up saying, "Yes, I know, but where do I find the time?" Well, start clocking how much time you spend on the Internet or watching TV and trust me, this little lie to yourself will be exposed pretty quickly.

There are ways to get busy without getting a gym membership you will never use. There are so many things in day that can all add up to make a difference – you just need to start and to keep on doing it! Here are just a few tips:

- Take the stairs – always. Don't do elevators, escalators or hot air balloons unless you must.
- Wake up every morning to a full stretch without even getting out of bed! Lie in bed and reach your arms up high over your head with feet pointed down. Start the stretch at your fingertips and work your way down to your toes. Try to feel every muscle pulling as you do it. Once fully extended, release the stretch just as slowly. The stretch should be 30 seconds long with the release another 30. Do it five times for one minute each.
- When standing in any line (grocery, bank, etc.) try to slowly lift one foot up two inches off the ground. Balance for 30 seconds and slowly put it down and then do the same with the other foot. This sounds a lot easier than it is and is a great way to tighten your rear.
- Walk whenever you can instead of driving. Park at the far back of the mall and walk to the entrance instead of taking 10 minutes to find the closest spot.
- While in your car, when you get to a red light sit up straight, shoulders rolled back and flex your stomach muscles (tighten and release) until you get the green.
- Every night do some try-to-touch-the-toes with the kids, grandkids or on your own. Remember, it is the trying that counts and stretch gently without rocking. Over time those toes will be staring you in the eye. Time for a pedi?
- Start listening to your breathing and to how your heart is responding to you, especially when doing something strenuous. By understanding your heartbeat and breathing you can get a better feel for how your body works. If the activity is too difficult, just slow down. If it is too easy to breathe, speed it up. Remember, it is YOU who is in control so listen to your body and change your actions accordingly.
- Breathe through stress with deep breaths to get the oxygen to your lungs and brain. Breathing can help your body feel energized and will get the oxygen you need to your cells.[45]

Once you have mastered a few of the daily steps to get your blood flowing and body awareness happening you can move on to the brisk walk and the aerobic routines to really get a jump start. Strive to get to 30 x 4 over time. Trust me – once you get in to the "move groove" you will not want to stop!

Also, remember that sweating is a good thing. This is your body's automatic air conditioner and is a means to cool you down. Embrace the sweat and be grateful for it, because it means your body is working and removing toxins at the same time. Wipe your face down and keep going, being aware of your breathing in order to monitor whether you should speed up or take it down a notch.

Remember, studies show that successful long-term weight loss maintainers (average weight loss of 30 kg for an average of 5.5 years) share common strategies, including eating a diet low in the bad fats, frequent self-monitoring of body weight and food intake and high levels of regular physical activity. Even better news is that once these successful maintainers have maintained their weight loss for two to five years, the chances of longer-term weight loss success greatly increases![46]

Summary

The standard quick-fix approach to weight loss is not only ineffective long term but on average will make you bigger and less healthy than when you began. Most weight gain takes place over time, so to think you can lose it without a commitment of time is simply unrealistic and downright silly. There is no drive-thru weight loss program that will work long-term.

To have lasting results, you need to take baby steps to reduce food consumption in order to keep your metabolism happy and healthy. Increasing energy-rich food alternatives, instead of the easy go-to of nutrient-poor processed and high-bad-fat foods, will allow your body to be even more engaged and ready to take on new challenges. With small but steady changes to increase your overall activity level, you will facilitate weight loss and have greater energy. So stand up, stretch and go!

What you know now:

- Diets DO NOT work over the long term.
- Changes to health and weight are long-term goals and must be realistic and done over time.
- Changing the type of food you eat and the amounts eaten, along with daily exercise is the only effective way of achieving long-term weight loss and overall health.

Apply to your daily routine:

- Commit to applying the daily food routines in this book.
- Keep high-protein, clean and unsweetened energy bars in your purse, glove compartment or briefcase.
- When your body is craving food, make sure it is healthy and energizing that way you will maintain energy levels and will want to move.
- Listen to your breathing and be aware of how your body is responding to your movements.
- Move. Just move! Start slowly and work up. Get into the "move groove" and your body will ask for more. Stick to it – you can do it!
- Once changes are part of your routine and you stabilize, add more challenging ones to get that extra bit better and move on to the next level.

Mind Chatter – What are your whispers saying?

Everyone is a moon and has a dark side which he never shows to anybody.
Mark Twain, author and humorist (1835-1910)

Since the ripe old age of fourteen, I smoked cigarettes: a lot of them. Initially I just thought it was cool, then I liked the taste and wanted more and eventually I couldn't stop. It took my Mom dying of lung cancer when I was 21 years old to motivate me to end this path of self-destruction and even then it took three years after her death for me to actually do it. I remember that just before I quit I asked a friend who had successfully weaned himself how he did it. He looked at me deadpan and said, "Just don't smoke." At the time, I thought he was such a fool.

But at 24 years of age, I woke up one morning and had a cigarette. I looked down and realized I had lit a second one from my still-lit first butt. It was 6:30 a.m. on a workday. Pathetic, I thought. I have to quit. So, after years of thinking about it and planning for some date in the future when I would, I quit cold turkey. Other than natural childbirth, it was one of the hardest things I have ever done. The VOICES! The conversations you have with the devil of addiction are scary, because you realize you have very little control. Once you decide to stop, you realize how much power this obsessive beast has on you as it controls your very being.

Needless to say, I have effectively kicked the habit (after a six-month period of falling off the nicotine wagon in my 30s), but I say that with a caveat of reality. I still have voices in my head that tell me to do it, especially when I am stressed out. I have a reoccurring dream in which I grab a smoke from some stranger and light it, but before I can take my first heavenly inhalation I awaken to the horrible truth that I am an ex-smoker in a well-ventilated bedroom.

But the voices and I have made a pact with the cancer-stick-demon and it is this: at 80 years of age I will start again. In fact, for my 80th birthday I want a pallet of smokes, a case of scotch and a pack or two of playing cards. Forget the bows and wrapping paper, just hand over the toxic goods and let me start again. I figure by then I will have lived a full, happy and healthy life so I can regress into old age happily sucking on noxious sticks and washing them down with moonshine until my bell tolls.

The reality is if I am lucky enough to get to 80 I will probably decide not to start up again ... but who cares? My delusional dream of my 80th gets me through the many well-ventilated nights with my voices droning on in the background.

Through breaking the habit, I became aware of how many other voices I have going on in my head. These voices or, as I like to call them, "whispers," are common ... you just don't know this because no one talks about it. Like the hundreds of thousands of women, myself included, who never admit to having miscarried due to feelings of shame and unwarranted grief, these phantom whispers become our crazy little secrets.

At one time or another, most of us fixate on something that distracts us from being happy and results in feelings of guilt, fear, failure, rejection, anxiety or depression. These fixations are often repetitive patterns of behaviour that you keep doing even though you know it is destructive. In an attempt to keep the behaviour "safe," you keep this info as your own furtive friend and don't discuss it but for the table tennis going on in your noggin'. Let me just say this: fixations and compulsive thoughts or behaviours are more common than not. If you have never had any them, you are truly an extraterrestrial and need to call your star base right about NOW to be beamed back to the mother ship, only to ditch this book prior to departure. For the rest of us struggling earth-bound humans, what are we to do?

If you compulsively use or do something despite its detrimental effects and crave it, then you have a dependency issue. However, there are many levels of dependency, some more extreme and damaging than others.[47] For the majority of us, our compulsions are usually self-damaging and centre on body image: binge eating, punitive eating (anorexia, bulimia) and dieting. In fact, our society's preoccupation with body image is so extensive that at any given time 70 per cent of women and 35 per cent of men are dieting.[48] More seriously, a 1993 Statistics Canada Survey reported that in women between the ages of 15 and 25, one to two per cent have anorexia and three to five per cent have bulimia. Eating disorders are not about food, but are a way of coping with deeper problems that are too painful or difficult to deal with directly. They cross all cultural, racial and socio-economic boundaries and affect men and women alike.[49]

But eating issues are often difficult to overcome, since food is such an integral part of our social lives and sustains life itself. Even though it is a wonderful gift from the heavens, food is also tied to many emotional triggers such as childhood, family issues, holidays and self-perceptions of body image in a size-fixated society.

Additionally, food often has many historical judgments attached to it. We are often taught at a young age that by "being good" we will get a food-based "treat." Likewise, certain foods may be taken away if we act poorly. We may have been told to eat everything on the plate even when we are full or dislike the taste. In adult life, we are bombarded with the conflicting images of media-worshipped skinny minis combined with ads for fast food and all-you-can-eat buffets and supersized options.

Such cultural teachings centre on a penalty and reward system that can manifest itself in poor eating habits and choices. For example, you may feel badly about yourself, so you overindulge as an attempt to provide an emotional means of filling a void. Or you may restrict your intake as a type of self-inflicted punishment and as a means of obtaining control. You may feel good about yourself and "over reward," as this is the pat on the back you need and find comfort in. All these choices are poor ones, but the behaviours are common and take place daily in many people's lives.

The good news is with a little self-understanding and a few tricks you can make it possible to get the control back. Only by understanding that something is controlling how you think, react and plan can you say, "Stop." But how?

Acknowledgement

The first step is acknowledgement. Listen to yourself and be aware of the conversations that go on in your head. Don't allow yourself to lie to YOU. Be aware of what little whispers are going on upstairs. What do you tell yourself to validate and excuse the poor choices you make? Once you know what this is, say it out loud. Saying it out loud will allow you to acknowledge it and stop hiding it in your own head. Even better, say it to someone else – then the cat is really out of the bag and you have to admit it is real. This will be a long process, but by catching yourself in these daily untruths you will be surprised at what an amazing liar you actually are!

Desire

The next step is to want to change so as to put those voices to rest. When I was younger and complaining one day about not having time to get to the gym, a friend said, "Half your workout is just to get there." What an idiot, I thought. But upon reflection and the wisdom of years, I think this is true. Half the battle of changing behaviour is acknowledging that the behaviour is not working for you and that you desire to make a difference. Only through acknowledgement and a desire to change will you be able to act in order to help rebuild the new you.

Origins

The next step is to understand the root of the behaviour. Dependency and compulsive behaviour are just misplaced emotions. For example, you binge eat not because you have a God-given need to pack it all in, but because you may feel angry or upset due to a previous event or trauma. But the trauma is not "front and centre" – it has manifested itself in a ritual of behaviour you now routinely follow. But it is the emotional reaction to the trauma that then plays itself out or expresses itself in your self-destructive choices and responses. By understanding the greater issue of the "why," you can figure out what the triggers are for your poor choices and either confront such triggers or avoid them altogether.

Stress

Managing stress levels is a major factor in reducing compulsive behaviour. For example, you could be on a great program of eating well and getting exercise and the second your mother-in-law comes to visit you fall off the wagon. Speaking of wagons, those chocolate-covered wagon wheels of childhood comfort suddenly call out your name at 2 a.m.![50] To make it even more stressful, your mother-in-law has beaten you to it and none are left. ARGH! Instead of giving in to the stress and letting it control you, try to confront it and work through it as a key part of avoiding the triggers of poor behaviour.

There are a number of ways to reduce stress and address the trauma of the past. An excellent tool is simply talking. Once articulated, the issue then steps outside your mind, because acknowledging it makes it real. Talk to trusted friends and family. I also highly endorse going to a professionally-trained therapist to work through things. Seeking help does not make you a "nut-case" or a "screw-ball." It is a smart decision and a great opportunity to have a professionally-trained person, who is objective and non-judgmental, get to the bottom of an issue and provide you with the coping tools to help you move past it. You can also take back control by initiating new positive routines that distract you from the previous destructive ones, which over time will "reprogram" your negative behaviour. Additionally and best of all, stress can be substantially reduced by getting some exercise, which makes you feel happy due to the endorphins released through aerobic activity. Adding exercise to your routine will increase your sense of power as you become physically stronger and more in control.

Time

Researchers now know that the brain needs about a 90-day "time-out" to reset itself, kind of like a computer that needs to be reprogrammed. By doing so, Yale University researchers found the brain was able to make proper decisions and analysis after this time. But if food is your demon of choice, it is impossible not to eat for 90 days in order to get a new hard drive.

Instead, take a small action every day for 90 days to reduce your destructive behaviour. You may not eliminate it altogether, but a reduction will start you on the path of better being. For example, if you eat ice cream every night, start by cutting the portion in half, then only eat it every other day, then switch to eating it only on Friday and Saturday nights. If you are aware of what your cravings are and take manageable steps that can be achieved, you can master those negative voices in your head.

Nurture your Mind and Body

Adding in new, simple routines to feed and nurture your body will also help. If you have emotional stress, your body will respond. By keeping your body healthy, alkaline and properly fed, your body can support you while your mind is dealing with its issues. It can be as simple as ensuring your body starts its day with a smile, by providing it with a nutrient-rich breakfast. Make time for a fruit and protein smoothie as an afternoon snack instead of a chocolate bar and add a tablespoon of seeds or nuts to your lunch sandwich or salad. By taking small steps to change your routine and by adding great super foods, your body will eventually feel the added energy and will be much more willing to take you back to positive behaviour that leaves you feeling better about yourself and will lead you down the road to wellness.

Summary

For those of us who are not aliens, we have all made bad choices and acted in a compulsive way at one time or another. Other than physical addictions, the behaviour hardest to overcome is the repetitive kind tied to negative emotions and food addictions or compulsions. The good thing is that this is common and you are not alone in this struggle. But by taking small steps and being aware of what you are thinking, why you are thinking it and how you choose to have it manifest in your daily choices and life you can make a difference and make some easy changes to get to a better you!

What you know now:

- Compulsive behaviour regarding food is not uncommon, so don't feel alone.
- Making poor choices can be very alienating, as you believe they are hidden from everyone. This can perpetuate negative feelings and result in behaviour that becomes a never-ending pattern.
- The key to changing your behaviour and to taking back control is to take steps to: (1) know you are doing it, (2) have a desire to change it, (3) reduce the emotional and situational triggers through identifying them and reducing exposure to them; (4) take manageable actions over time to make a difference and (5) start a new and simple food routine that is positive and energy-adding.

Apply to your daily routine:
- Be aware of the lies you tell yourself. The only person you are fooling is you. Instead, live in your own real world: ask yourself questions, listen to your answers, understand your reasons … and repeat (∞).
- Set a conscious and achievable goal regarding which voices you want to shut down. Make a 90-day plan to reduce the negative behaviour by taking small daily actions to reduce the triggers for poor behaviour. Set manageable goals you can implement to attain your 90-day plan. Chart your changes daily on a calendar in the kitchen. Then once achieved, set a new goal.
- Get some good old exercise to reduce stress – it will make a big difference and will help to diffuse the poor pattern triggers.
- Talk to trusted friends and family and engage them to help and support you. Seek professional help if and when you need it – we all do at some point. I highly recommend it!
- Add in some great foods daily to help you start some new good-for-you routines and get you off the pattern of penalty.

Stress Reduction

Anxiety is fear of one's self.
Wilhelm Stekel, Austrian psychologist (1868-1940)

Other than caring for my mom during her fight against cancer and the horrible aftermath that ensued, I have had a couple of hugely stressful moments in my life. One of them was the second time firefighters came to our newly-purchased farmhouse.

As I mentioned in the preface, in an attempt to lead a better life for our children and ourselves, my husband and I decided to say goodbye to city life and head for the hills. We sold off all we had and moved to a 100-acre farm an hour and half north of the city in order to get back to the basics. Gone was the nanny, gone were the private schools, gone was the corporate life and gone was the stress of living in a 24/7 chaotic world of traffic and break-ins.

After moving to our farmhouse during the cold month of November, my friend and I worked feverishly to get the place perfect. Four days later, almost everything was unpacked, the pictures were hung and the place looked incredible. I had thought of everything ... or so I thought.

What happened next was that it got cold. I dread being cold. I quickly realized that I had truly underestimated the draftiness of a farmhouse built in 1860. What were these penny-pinching pilgrims thinking by not installing insulation? I was freezing and the gas furnace obviously wasn't working as well as hoped due to various external doors that didn't fit their hinges and an uninsulated basement. I caved in and lit the kitchen woodstove without first having it cleaned. What could happen with only one fire? Apparently, a lot.

The following afternoon, after the cozy fire of the night before was long gone, my visiting sister gave me a blast for having left the fire extinguishers too close to the woodstove's exhaust brick chimney stack that went from the basement up into the country kitchen, into the second floor bedroom and out of the roof. "They could have exploded!" she said sternly. What? I touched the brick and it was scorching hot to the touch ... but the woodstove fire had been out for more than 12 hours! My heart sank and I ran out the front door. I looked at the outside chimney and saw smoke and I knew it was trouble. "I think we have a chimney fire," I yelled to my husband. Like a scene out of a bad movie, I kept yelling, "Call 911!"

Over four hours later the three fire truck pumpers finally left our house, taking with them the 30 firefighters who had been running all over our lawn and roof and in our house, the police who were directing traffic and the local news crew who filmed our fire to broadcast to the world what happens when you act like an idiot and do not clean your fireplace. The fire chief told us if we had waited any longer to call them, our house would likely be completely lost. In its wake we had a wall ripped down, water pumped through our chimney (which resulted in a horrific smell throughout our house) and the need to rip out our old chimney and purchase a new woodstove.

We are so lucky! I thank my lucky stars and the fire department for our lives and our beautiful home. The firefighters were unbelievable (even sweeping and mopping up the mess). My respect for firefighters continues but, honestly, I hope they keep their distance and I really don't want to see another one up close for quite some time.

That night we went to bed at 10 p.m., contemplating how truly blessed we were. At 1:30 a.m. I bolted up in bed in the midst of a full-on anxiety attack. I could not breath, I could not stop sweating and my ears felt like they were going to explode. The thought that I could have killed my children and other loved ones due to my neurotic need to be warm was overwhelming. I was completely paralyzed and incapable of shutting down. No matter what I did, I could not rid my mind of the negative thoughts swirling around in my head. At the end of my sleepless night, I eagerly welcomed the light of day because I had an excuse to get up and distract myself with the clean up. I was experiencing a mild case of post-traumatic stress disorder. It took me more than a week to feel like I was once again living in reality.

Mental stress is an incredibly powerful emotion that often manifests itself in physical conditions. Conversely, it can also be a physical condition due to poor nutrition that leads to physical and emotional responses. For example, if you eat a diet high in refined foods, your body will have to make the additional effort to try to rebalance itself, creating stresses internally that will leave you feeling lethargic and tired. Symptoms of stress on any level include fatigue, poor sleep, caffeine dependence and low energy.

Stress is like a fire: when controlled and used for a purpose, it serves us well as it did when our ancestors had to forage and survive in the wild. Additionally, certain stresses are beneficial, like exercise. When you exercise and then rest, your body will eventually grow stronger. But with today's increased levels of stress, with less physical means to release it, this fire left unbridled can be all consuming.

In his book *The Thrive Diet*, Brendan Brazier outlines how the body responds to stress, both beneficially and negatively. In either case, cortisol (sometimes referred to as the "stress hormone") is released as a result of physical or psychological stress. Because of the release of cortisol in reaction to the onset of stress, your body actually gains energy. You will become more alert, your strength may increase and you will be able to process information more quickly and react slightly faster than usual. Much like my heightened sense of being in the moment while watching and waiting to see if our house would burn down! However, without a period of rest, cortisol will eventually eat away at your body by breaking down muscle tissue.[51]

Stress has a spiraling effect on your body. In a desperate attempt to re-metabolize after chronic stress, your body goes into a kind of perpetual state of shock. From stress, you have fatigue. If left unchecked, the body shifts fuel sources from fat to carbs and your body begins to store fat, resulting in your body craving carbs. By eating more carbs you end up producing more stress, because your body has to work even harder as it gets fatter and less efficient.

To avoid the downward stress spiral, superior energy-maximizing foods offer the greatest source of sustainable energy. Avoid caffeine and highly-refined sugars, which only result in quick bouts of stimulation. As Brendan points out, "High net-gain whole foods provide a platform on which to build long-term sustainable vitality."[52]

What is so great about this? Your body perceives not eating enough nutrient-rich foods as being stressful, so by eating more high-dense quality foods there are situations when eating more will reduce your body-fat percentage! The bottom line is that nutrient-rich whole foods have nutritional stress reduction properties, which can help you get a better sleep and attain your ideal body weight. Eating good food reduces the body's physical stress and can help reduce the body's physical responses to mental stress.

Some means of reducing mental stresses include:

Consciously Breathe

Inhale deeply, drawing the breath down into the pit of your stomach while filling your lungs and then hold it for five seconds and release. Do this for as long as needed to feel de-stressed. By drawing in air through to the lower lung (versus the common means of doing short breaths that only reach the upper lung) you will regain control, draw in greater oxygen, slow your blood rate, decrease blood pressure and relieve anxiety. Studies indicate that deep breathing has incredible healing abilities and can significantly reduce symptoms of severe PMS, anxiety and depression.[53]

Voice Anxiety

Acknowledge the real reason why you are anxious and say it out loud. If you feel adversarial towards your spouse and yell at the kids, reflect and understand why. Is the source of your anger due to your hubby and offspring or is it really the anxiety about that day's important meeting? When you say it out loud ("I am nervous about the meeting.") either to yourself or a close confidant you immediately acknowledge the root cause of your anxiety. Understanding the source of the stress can help to relieve it and lessen your likelihood of blaming any bystanders (including yourself!).

Address Control

Be aware of how much control you can exercise over the situation, either by taking action (control) or letting it go (no control). For example, if you are convinced the world is ending, there's not much you can do about it. To worry about this takes energy you could be using to enjoy yourself. However, if you are worried the planet is at risk as a result of pollution or global warming, you can take measures in your daily life to counteract its environmentally-damaging effects and take action to create change. In one scenario, you have no control, so let it go and live life to the fullest. In the second example, you do have control so take charge and get actively involved. Likewise, address control over feelings of guilt as it can be a huge source of stress and is toxic to your body. If something has already happened, you can't change the event. But you do have control over your response to it and acceptance of it. Do what you have to do to let go: apologize if you need to, forgive others and yourself, and move on. Changing your perception of a problem is often the core to finding a solution to it.

Move for Stress Management

Aerobic activity is a great way to relieve stress and stay healthy. You don't really need any more than 30 minutes of activity four times a week to ensure you remain healthy. To be really fit you will need to spend more time exercising, but at a minimum the 30 x 4 rule is a good one. Remember this does not have to be spent in a gym or done all at once. The important thing is to get your body moving as part of your weekly routine.

If you do an activity that you enjoy, you will continue with it rather than feel like you have embarked upon a torture program. The bottom line is to have fun and shake your chakras!!! Do something you love and just keep it up – the odds are more likely you will stick to it. Also, you won't cause your body unneeded stress by trying to make something happen that just doesn't fit into your busy world.

The Top 10 Ways

To get moving there are some simple steps you can take to get on the right path. To give you some ideas, I have set up my top 10 easiest and cheapest ways to get fit:

1. Sex

You have to love something that feels great, costs no money and will help slim you down. A woman weighing 160 pounds having five minutes of foreplay and 20 minutes of sex loses approx 110 calories. Not only is sex a great exercise, but orgasms also release endorphins that make you feel happy and positive about yourself! So have a good roll (safe sex always) to get a good workout in and feel perky.

2. Walk

Simple and cheap, this is a great way to get in some quality time with your partner, friends or kids or just have some you time. You can get in a cardiovascular workout without even breaking a sweat! A person weighing 62kg (or 137 pounds) and walking an hour at an average speed will burn about 260 calories. Not a bad return for a walk and talk! So grab a walking partner and make it part of your daily routine.

3. Super(wo)man

This one is super easy, can be done anywhere and brings relief to your back while strengthening it. Lie down on your stomach on the floor with your eyes looking at the floor. Point your toes downwards and elongate your body to get a good stretch in. While holding the stretch, bring your arms out in front of you (raised about four inches from the ground) and point your thumbs up towards the ceiling. Take a deep breath, pull back your shoulders and start to slowly raise your arms towards the ceiling while bringing your shoulders and then your chest off the ground. At the same time, slowly raise both legs up off the ground. Your arms and feet should both be heading for the ceiling at the same time – strive to have your body looking like a semicircle. Squeeze your bum muscles and exhale and slowly return to starting position. Repeat as many times as you can but aim for 20 a day to get good returns. If this is too tricky with both arms and legs then simply alternate between opposite arm and leg. Make sure you avoid jerking your neck and you don't tuck your head into your shoulders.

4. Wall Push-ups

This is an easy way to get the benefits of push-ups without the pain of doing it on the floor. I could never do a full push-up even at the height of my "fit self" because it always hurt my toes. Pick any wall and stand facing it with your toes two feet away. Extend your arms out and place your hands, shoulder width apart, on the wall in front of you. Keep your body straight and pull in your abdominal muscles. Bending only at the elbows, slowly lower yourself forward towards the wall. Then slowly push yourself away from it. Pick a spot in your home that you walk past frequently and plan to stop and do one every time you walk past that spot. You won't believe how much of a difference this one makes. Aim for 20 a day.

5. Squats

This one is easy – if you do a couple every time you are about to sit down for a meal you will be fit in no time! Grab a kitchen chair and stand about 1.5 feet away from it. Place your hands on top of chair. Point your feet towards the chair and keep them shoulder width apart. Keep your torso straight, abdominal muscles tight and slightly arch your back. Slowly bend your knees while keeping them over your toes. Squat down as far as it is comfortable, hold the position and then slowly raise yourself by using your leg muscles. Do 20 a day.

6. Standing Calf Raises

This one is a great way to get nice summer legs and have them year-round. Pick some stairs or get out an old thick phone book. Stand on the edge of the step/book with only the balls of your feet on the step/book. Keeping your knees stiff, body straight and tall, lower your heels down slowly towards the floor. Only bend at the ankle. Go down as far as you can until you feel a strong stretch in your calves. Aim for 20 a day. Reverse the direction – don't bounce – and then push up on the balls of your feet as high as you can. Start by doing both feet at the same time and then go to one foot for greater challenge. Do this while talking on the phone and you can get your workout in without even thinking about it.

7. Arm Twirls

This one requires a bit of room, but is a great way to get tighter arms and get an upper back workout. Stand straight with your tummy tight and your feet shoulder width apart. Extend both arms out at shoulder height with fingers pointed straight. Start to make small circles the size of a doughnut (the one you will never eat again) in a clockwise motion. Speed up your circles and do 50 of them. Then reverse and do them counter clockwise. After completing the doughnut-sized ones, start to make huge circles (the size of a bike tire – the one you will soon be riding everywhere) clockwise and then reverse. You will have a toned upper back and arms in no time!

8. Just Sit There

This is the easiest thing you can ever do to stay fit and aligned. Whenever you are sitting (at work, in a car or in front of the TV or computer) make sure you do the following:

- Keep your shoulders back, not rolled forward. This will keep your chest muscles stretched out and your neck and upper back as well.
- Sit upright. This will force your lower back to stretch and will give your abs a little stretch as well. During every set of commercials on TV or every 15 minutes at your desk or in the car, contract your ab muscles; release and repeat 20 times. This will give you more success than doing sit-ups once a week.
- Raise your heels off the ground and go up and down with your heels quickly so as to jiggle your entire leg. This will keep circulation going and will exercise your leg muscles. P.S.: don't do the "jiggles" while driving the car – only as a passenger!

9. Balance

During any "unused moments" like waiting in line, waiting for public transit or talking on the phone, balance on one foot and raise the other off the ground 1 inch or more and balance for 30 seconds. Alternate your feet. This will help to develop your core strength and is a great way to exercise in lost time. Do this 10 times for each foot.

10. Laugh!

Research indicates laughter can be the best medicine for weight loss. While studying adults watching film clips, the researchers discovered that laughing increased the heart rate and calorie expenditure of all participants by up to 20 per cent! The longer they laughed, the greater the effects. Using the results, the researchers calculated that with 15 minutes of laughter a day you can burn 10 to 40 calories (depending on the laughter's intensity and the person's weight), which is enough to lose a couple of pounds a year. So keep on laughing!

Summary

Stress is not necessarily a bad thing and can be a huge benefit to your physical well-being. But when stress is not useful to you, it is important to quickly identify it in order to set up parameters for dealing with it. If not effectively dealt with, this uncomplimentary source of stress will affect you negatively both mentally and physically and if left unchecked will result in disease and illness.

Stress is like a bottled genie and has to be let out in order to confront it. Acknowledgement of stressful triggers combined with exercise to physically release it, are the best means to get things under control.

What you know now:
- Stress is a powerful emotion and leads to a physical response that can have a huge impact on your well-being.
- Although it can be a positive influence, it is important to reduce negative stress levels.
- Poor food choices also affect your mental health and your body's physically stressed response.

Apply to your daily routine:
- Breathe! Take deep breathes upon arising in the morning and at bedtime to increase oxygen levels. Breathe deeply through any trauma or stress to ensure your body is given the nutrients to cope. Remember, life is just a series of continuous breaths.
- Make better food choices that reduce stress on the body. Every day, aim for five to eight whole food portions that are easily digestible and include all three food pillars.
- Get better sleep by having an active day physically combined with good food choices (especially your last meal of the day). Ensure you get enough magnesium daily in your diet as this greatly assists in sleepy time.

Functional Foods

. . . .

There is no love more sincere than the love of food.
George Bernard Shaw, playwright (1856-1950)

My ex-mother-in-law is a wonderful woman. She is a first genera-
tion Italian and I learned a lot about regional Italian cooking
as a result of her knowledge and patience. One dish she taught
me to make was my favourite and no matter how many times I made it,
it never tasted as delicious as hers. Thinking I was missing some key in-
gredient, I asked her what it was. She smiled and placed each one of her
well-worn hands on either side of my face and said in her lovely rich accent,
"Anna, that is because I make mine with my love – and that is what you
are tasting." I thought this was the most incredible concept and after years
of contemplation, I believe it to be true.

As you know, there is no comparison between the homemade soup of one
who loves you, rather one whipped up by an unknown cook and delivered
to your restaurant table by a hardworking mortal who wants a good tip!
Likewise, the tea and toast your mom makes for you when you are sick
can never be replicated by your own hands, no matter how high your self-
esteem is that day. Vegetables grown by someone's caring hand can never
be simulated by those bought from the grocery store. There is something
so magical and mystical about food grown and made with love – the food

itself serves as a symbol of the "sustenance of the soul" we wish to endow upon those we adore. But when food is lacking this care and this valuable essence, can it also have the opposite effect? I truly believe that it can.

Although raised in a vegetarian household, our six-year-old son really wants to eat meat. He knows it and expresses it constantly. My husband and I decided to let him make that choice for himself but on two conditions: any meat he eats must be organic/free-range and when eating it he must acknowledge it gave its life for him. In a world of fast food and convenience, many forget the nicely wrapped and packaged hamburgers in the grocery freezer or bloodless chicken breast wrapped in non-recyclable packaging is an animal … an animal that gave its life in order for you to consume it. My belief is if you are going to eat it, then make sure the animal was well-cared for and died with little pain and suffering, because that trauma is what you are ultimately putting into your body. In addition, there is the taste factor. If you are a meat eater, I urge you to source an organic butcher, spend a couple of extra dollars and buy a piece of organic free-range meat. There is a world of difference in taste.

The same is true of fruits and vegetables. Like the food grown in a green-thumb's summer backyard, there is nothing that compares to an organic and pesticide-free fruit or veggie. In fact, before I had eaten an organic grapefruit I never liked them. As soon as I tried an organic one my mouth lit up like the Times Square Christmas tree. The difference in taste is really amazing. Additionally, you know you are not storing any toxins as a result of eating what is supposed to be good for you! What is the point of eating blueberries for their antioxidant factor when they are covered in carcinogenic pesticides? You know, our culture really is nutty sometimes.

Another benefit I have noticed from eating organic food is I don't need as much to feel happy and full – it does the trick the first time around. My ugly small organic apple gives me a much greater energy boost and tastes better than the lovely looking (but nasty tasting) big shiny one sitting in the basket at the end of the coffee counter. Although organics are more expensive, at the end of the day I need to buy less food, so it really does balance out any out-of-pocket pennies.

The other environmental benefit of free range and organic choices is that most are locally-grown and the farms are family-run. This translates into a smaller footprint for the food to get to your table, which means you are reducing the amount of pollution produced to allow you to sit down for your supper. If local farmers are supported it will also, over time, decrease the cost of the food and will ensure nutrient-rich soil continues to be farmable for future generations.

Just to be clear, organic is simply a fancy word made up for what our fore-fathers and fore-mothers already knew and did on their family-operated farms. There is nothing new in this, only a tagline based on a pretty simple concept: keep your food pollutant-free (pesticides, herbicides, genetically modified) so you don't digest the toxins or contaminate the soil for yourself or your lineage.

To summarize, the following is a snapshot of the benefits of choosing organic produce, organic dairy and free-range meats:
- Reduces the toxins you have in your system.
- Ensures you have better energy in your food so you are digesting the care and respect put into it.
- Supports your local and family-run farming community to enable them to grow and continue to provide food to your area.
- Means you eat and buy less food because you need less, as nutrient-rich foods give greater sustenance with less caloric intake required.
- Promotes environmentally-supportive farming practices.

A cheap alternative to organic and free-range foods is to go direct to the farmers and buy in bulk – this will cut out the middleman costs. Another cost-effective means of opting for organic alternatives is to join a cooperative food group that focuses on natural and organic options. You can also source local organic farms, go to local farmers' markets in season, freeze produce for winter wants and look into organic produce delivery services in your area. The best option of all is to start a garden in your own backyard and grow it yourself! Remember, if you cannot afford all organics at your table, ensure you choose organic produce for fruits and veggies that absorb the most toxins, those with no skin (salad greens, celery), thin skins (apples, peppers, etc.) or ground grown (root veggies, potatoes, etc.).

Food Fill-osophy

To get the best results, you must talk to your vegetables.
Charles, Prince of Wales (b.1948)

I have chosen these recipes with care. In my world, food has to be really tasty, as I want all the calories to be worth it. It has to be relatively easy to prepare (meaning I don't have to find an obscure cultural marketplace to buy the ingredients, nor buy a new serving dish or cooking contraption in order to make it). Lastly, it has to be healthy. With all this in mind, I have created these recipes.

As you now know, a plant-based diet is the best choice to substantially reduce health risks and increase your body's functionality. But you can easily get better by incorporating more fruits, veggies and nuts into your daily routine and by reducing any dairy and meat reliance over time. To this end I have created theses recipes without dairy, fish or meat. But feel free to add them if and where it makes sense. To make it a little easier, I have also added some optional suggestions.

Have fun with these recipes and add and subtract ingredients as your creative juices require – but I think these recipes will provide you with a great starting point to become a little bit better.

Bon Appétit!

Recipes

Fun Food

I love to serve dips as they instantly create a communal, shared experience. Instead of the traditional dips high in the bad fats, the following four dips offer nutritious taste-infused solutions rich in protein, vitamins and essential fatty acids. Don't tell the kids or friends that these are good for them – they won't believe you anyway! The base for the dips is all the same so have some fun and experiment with your favourite flavours.

Banana Dip

Kids love this one, as it tastes great and they can "play" with their food. Serve with pieces of different types of fresh fruit to add to the fun and nutrition.

> 1 cup commercially-roasted hemp seeds
> ¼ cup brown rice milk
> 2 tbsp olive oil
> 1 ripe banana
> ½ tsp cinnamon
> ½ tsp vanilla
> 2 tbsp maple syrup
> ¼ tsp dried ginger
> pinch of nutmeg

Blend first three ingredients in food processor until smooth. Add remaining ingredients and blend until smooth.

Tabouli Dip

This is a new take on an old favourite. The parsley and tomato give this dip a fresh taste and the chickpeas offer up a smooth finish. Coupled with whole grain pita, the chickpeas add to the hemp seeds' protein power and combine to make a complete protein.

1 cup commercially-roasted hemp seeds
¼ cup brown rice milk
2 tbsp olive oil
2 tbsp lemon juice
¼ tsp ground black pepper
1 ⅓ cups washed and patted dry fresh chopped parsley
1 plum tomato chopped with most seeds removed
2 small garlic cloves
⅔ cup cooked and drained chickpeas
2 tsp onion powder
½ tsp sea salt (optional)
½ tsp tandoori seasoning or ground cumin

Blend first three ingredients in food processor until smooth. Add remaining ingredients and blend until smooth.

Serve with whole grain pita or vegetable sticks.

Cilantro Avocado Dip

This dip has a lively taste and is even better when combined with whole grain tortilla chips or slices of whole grain pita. The cilantro is chock full of chlorophyll and fibre and is a good source of iron, magnesium and mangelese. The avocado and hemp seeds provide rich good fats.

1 cup commercially-roasted hemp seeds
¼ cup brown rice milk
2 tbsp olive oil
¼ cup washed and patted dry chopped cilantro
2 tbsp lime juice
1 small clove garlic
1 tsp chili powder
1 plum tomato diced with seeds removed
1 ripe and diced avocado
½ tsp sea salt (optional)
1 dash of hot sauce (optional)
½ cup shredded cheddar cheese (optional)

Blend first three ingredients in food processor until smooth. Add remaining ingredients and blend until desired consistency.

Lentil Curry Dip

This dip has a rich, complex and mildly spicy taste. It is full of hemp seed protein and has even more complete proteins when combined with whole grain breads or crackers due to the amount of red lentils.

    1 cup commercially-roasted hemp seeds
    ¼ cup brown rice milk
    2 tbsp olive oil
    1 cup cooked red lentils
    ½ heaping tsp ground cumin
    ½ heaping tsp ground coriander
    ½ tsp chili powder
    ¼ tsp tumeric
    ¼ tsp dried ground ginger
    ¼ tsp cinnamon
    1 pinch nutmeg
    1 garlic clove
    4 tbsp orange juice
    2 tsp onion powder

Blend first three ingredients in food processor until smooth. Add remaining ingredients and blend until desired consistency.

Stuffed Mushrooms

Mushrooms are very high in some key antioxidants, which studies indicate may help prevent breast cancer. The high amount of niacin in mushrooms may also help to prevent or delay Alzheimer's and other cognitive disorders. Other nutrients and minerals found in mushrooms include iron, potassium and zinc. While munching on these delicious appetizers, know that there is no downside to eating them, especially the non-dairy version!

1 ½ tbsp Salba whole seeds
1 tsp olive oil
1 tsp hemp oil
1 tsp balsamic vinegar
454 g box of white or brown mushrooms
1 tsp olive oil
3 green onions, minced (about ⅔ cup)
3 tbsp washed and patted dry minced parsley
½ tsp sea salt
1 tsp paprika
1 tsp onion powder
½ tsp garlic powder
2 tbsp commercially-roasted or regular hemp seeds
¼ cup parmesan or ½ cup shredded mozzarella cheese (optional)

Preheat oven to 325°F. Combine first four ingredients and mix together in a bowl. Wash and clean the mushrooms well. With a paring knife, remove the stems of the mushroom along with a rounded ridge and place in a separate small bowl. The mushroom caps should now have a small cavity – set them aside. Take the stems/ridges and finely chop.

In a fry pan, add olive oil on medium/high heat. Once heated, add mushroom stems/ridges and cook, stirring occasionally for about 10 minutes – until soft and with little water remaining. Add green onion and all other ingredients (excluding hemp seeds and cheese) and cook on medium heat for 10 minutes, stirring occasionally. Remove from heat, add hemp seeds and stir. Use mixture to gently stuff the mushroom caps. Add cheese on top if desired. Place on a lightly greased pan and bake for 25-30 minutes, until mushroom caps are browned. Makes about 15-20 mushroom caps.

Corn Fritters

Corn is a great, low-fat source of insoluble fibre and folic acid. This recipe is a great way to use up leftover corn on the cob or make a fast snack with frozen corn. Kids love these and they can also be served as snacks or appetizers.

2 tbsp Salba whole seeds
6 tbsp water
2 cups cooked corn kernels
2 tbsp commercially-roasted hemp seeds or regular hemp seeds
¾ tsp taco powder seasoning or chili powder
¼ tsp ground pepper
½ tsp garlic powder
1 tsp finely chopped washed and dried cilantro or parsley
1 tbsp onion powder
⅓ cup spelt flour or flour of your choice

Preheat oven to 325° F. Soak Salba in the water for 20 minutes to hydrate. Add cilantro to Salba mixture and stir. Mix dry ingredients together. Add corn and Salba/cilantro mixture to dry mixture and mix well. Press into 12 well-greased muffin tins. Pat down tops with spoon. Bake for 40 minutes. Use a knife to gently loosen sides and pop out with spoon. These can be served hot or cold and are best with a dab of salsa on the side.

All-Day Granola

This granola is a great make-ahead recipe and is easy on the pocketbook. It tastes great and is so loaded with nutrients you will want to eat it at every meal or snack time!

Step 1:
>   3 cups rolled oats (not instant)
>   ½ cup slivered unroasted almonds
>   ⅓ cup raw sunflower seeds
>   ⅓ cup raw pumpkin seeds
>   ½ tablespoon ground cinnamon
>   1 ½ tbsp melted coconut oil
>   ½ tsp vanilla
>   ½ cup agave nectar or maple syrup

Step 2:
>   ¼ cup Salba whole seeds
>   ½ cup commercially-roasted hemp seeds
>   ½ tbsp melted coconut oil
>   1 cup dried fruit (optional)

Preheat oven to 325° F. Mix together the first four Step 1 ingredients. In another bowl, stir together the coconut oil, vanilla, cinnamon and agave nectar (or maple syrup). Pour Step 1 wet mixture over Step 1 dry mixture and mix together until dry mixture is coated. Spread onto a pre-greased or parchment-paper-covered baking sheet. Bake in oven for approximately 25 minutes, stirring frequently. Remove from oven and decrease temperature to 300° F. Mix together all Step 2 ingredients (hemp seeds, Salba and remaining coconut oil) in a bowl and sprinkle on top of lightly baked oats mixture. Return baking sheet to oven for another ten minutes, until golden brown. Once browned, take out of the oven, stir and let cool on the baking sheet. Once cool, add 1 cup of dried fruit if you opt for it. Store in an airtight container in fridge. Makes about five cups.

Hearty Helpings

Split Pea & Orange Soup

This recipe makes about eight servings but is worth the extra work as it freezes so nicely. Cut the recipe in half it if you would like to have less of it.

2 ⅓ cups dry yellow split peas (or a 450 g package)
2 ⅓ cups dry green split peas (or a 450 g package)
2 tbsp olive oil
2 large cooking onions, diced (approximately 3 cups)
3 medium sweet potatoes or yams, peeled and diced into ½ inch pieces (approximately 5 cups)
⅛ tsp pepper
3 tbsp onion powder
3 tbsp maple syrup
1 cup orange juice
¼ tsp nutmeg
7 cups vegetable broth
½ cup commercially-roasted hemp seeds
Salt to taste

Place peas in cold water so it covers them plus one inch above. Soak split peas for three to six hours, then rinse well and set aside. If using canned ones, soaking is not required. Heat olive oil in large pot on medium/high heat. Add onions and stir frequently until light brown. Add in sweet potatoes and stir. Then add all peas and stir. Add six cups of the vegetable stock (leave the 7th cup aside) and the remaining ingredients, except the hemp seeds. Place on medium/low heat and cook for 30 minutes or until all beans are soft. Add the last cup of broth and add hemp seeds. Blend all ingredients in a food processor or with a wand blender until smooth. Serve with whole grain toasted bread or a side of brown rice.

Mushroom, Oat & Onion Soup

It may seem strange to put oats in a soup but this really tastes incredible. Plus, steel cut oats are gluten-free and full of protein and fibre. Miso – a traditional Japanese thick salty paste made from fermented rice, barley and soy beans – is high in protein, vitamins and minerals such as zinc, manganese and copper. The alkaline maca powder is high in fibre, calcium and vitamins B1, B2 and B12 and helps to boost energy, adding a powerful smoky punch to this rich and meaty-tasting soup.

3 cups water
1 cup uncooked steel cut oats (or pearled barley)
2 tbsp olive oil
2 medium red onions (approximately 2 cups)
10 green onions, chopped (approximately 2 cups)
6 medium Portobello mushrooms, chopped and stems removed (approximately 6 cups)
454g box sliced white mushrooms (approximately 6 cups)
1 cup water
4 cups vegetable stock
4 tsp maca powder (if you don't have, add 1 tsp at a time of powdered veggie soup base to taste)
4 tsp white or yellow miso paste
Parmesan cheese to taste (optional)

Boil three cups of water, place steel cut oats in water and simmer on medium/low for 15 minutes, stirring occasionally. Remove from element and cover. In a separate pot, heat olive oil over medium/high heat. Add diced red onion and cook for five minutes, stirring occasionally. Add green onions and cook for 10 minutes, stirring occasionally. Then add both kinds of mushrooms with the one cup of water, stir, cover and turn to low heat and cook for 10 minutes. Add the previously-cooked steel cut oats (or barley), vegetable stock, maca and miso and simmer for 20 minutes. Sprinkle with parmesan cheese if desired. Serves four as a main dish or six as an appetizer.

Mango Choco Chili

This chili makes the transition from stand-by staple to exotic main meal with the addition of mangos and cocoa to create sweet and sultry flavours. Cocoa is an excellent antioxidant and mangos are high in phenols (antioxidant properties) with vitamin E, vitamin A and selenium (an essential trace mineral).

2 tbsp olive oil
1½ cups diced white cooking onion (1 medium)
½ orange pepper, diced
½ red pepper, diced
1 ripe mango, peeled and diced (approximately 1¼ cups)
2-14 oz cans of unstrained diced tomato
(or 3 cups diced Roma tomatoes)
19 oz can of black beans, drained and rinsed
½ tsp salt
¼ tsp ground cumin
2 tsp chili powder
2 tsp maple syrup
2 tsp unsweetened cocoa powder
1 pinch ground cayenne pepper
1 tbsp commercially-roasted hemp seeds
1 tbsp Salba seeds

Heat olive oil on medium/high heat in a pot and add onion. Stir occasionally and cook until onions are lightly browned. Add peppers and mango. Reduce heat to medium and sauté until peppers sweat, approximately five minutes. Add tomatoes and beans and stir. Add all other ingredients, reduce to low and let simmer about 10 minutes. Serves four as a main dish.

Extra option: Serve as a super healthy salsa by adding 2 tbsp of nutrient-rich Salba seeds. Mix and let cool for two hours before serving.

Thai Curry Soup

This seems like a lot of ingredients but many of these are easily obtained at most grocery stores and are likely already in your fridge or cupboard. There are also the less preferable pre-cut and frozen vegetable options or tube herb versions when you are in a rush. Feel free to add a cup of any additional veggie/meat protein. This is even better the next day, so leftovers are welcome!

Base:

2-400 ml cans coconut milk

4 cups vegetable broth

3 large basil leaves, minced

1 tbsp fresh lime juice

1 tsp store bought lemon grass puree or 1 tsp lemon zest

1 ½ tsp minced washed and dried cilantro

1 small wedge (½"x ½") of fresh ginger sliced into slim pieces or 1 ½ tsp ground ginger

½ tsp garlic powder

1 tsp onion powder

1 tsp Braggs soy amino acid (or soya sauce)

1-2 tsp mild curry paste (use ½ tsp if cooking for "spice-fearing" children like mine)

Veggies:

14 oz can miniature cob on corn, drained and rinsed (approximately 2 cups)

454 g box sliced white or brown mushrooms (approximately 6 cups)

½ head broccoli, sliced (approximately 1 ½ cups)

1 celery stick, diced (approximately 1 cup)

1 large carrot, diced (approximately 1 cup)

1 medium tomato, diced (approximately 1 cup)

2 green onions, chopped (approximately ½ cup)

Note: If you are in a rush, put in seven cups of frozen stir fry vegetables instead of the corn, mushrooms, broccoli, celery, carrot, and tomato.

1 cup roasted cashews

¼ cup commercially-roasted hemp seeds

Mix together all base ingredients to a cooking pot. Boil on medium/high heat for 15 minutes. Reduce to medium heat and add all veggies, except for cashews and hemp seeds and cook for 15 minutes. Reduce to simmer for 10 minutes. Take out 2 cups of soup liquid and add to a blender with cashews and hemp seeds. Blend until creamy and add back to soup, stir and serve! Makes six servings.

Rosemary Chickpea Special

This is so simple, yet tasty and easy to reheat. The tomatoes are a great anti-oxidant and the chickpeas combined with brown rice allow for a complete protein that is nutrient-dense and light on the pocketbook.

> 2 tbsp olive oil
> 2 medium white cooking onions, diced or ½ large Spanish onion, diced (approximately 2 cups)
> 3 cloves garlic minced
> 1 tsp dried rosemary
> 2 cups cooked chickpeas (approximately 1 can or 19 fl oz)
> 2-14 oz cans diced tomato
> 1 ½ tbsp Salba whole seeds
> Parmesan or Romano cheese to taste (optional)

In a medium saucepan, sauté onions and garlic in olive oil on medium heat until light brown (caramelized). Add rosemary, chickpeas and diced tomato and cook for another five minutes. Add Salba and cover and simmer on low heat for 20 minutes. Serve over brown rice with, optionally, a tablespoon of grated Parmesan cheese or Romano and freshly ground black pepper. Makes four servings.

Zingy Apple & Butternut Squash Soup

This beta-carotene and vitamin C-rich soup will become a favourite. Its rich and hearty taste will make this a sure fire winner with the whole family.

2 tbsp olive oil
3 medium white onions peeled and diced (approximately 4 cups)
1 medium butternut squash peeled and diced (approximately 8 cups)
3 medium apples peeled and diced (approximately 2 cups)
3 medium carrots peeled and diced (approximately 2 cups)
1 cup orange juice
½ tsp plus a pinch dried chili flakes
½ tsp plus a pinch ground allspice
½ tsp plus a pinch ground cinnamon
¼ tsp ground pepper (optional)
¾ tsp dried thyme
4 cups vegetable stock
1 cup commercially-roasted hemp seeds
6 tbsp low-fat sour cream (optional)

Add olive oil to stock pot and turn heat on medium/high. When heated, add onion and sauté until onions sweat and are light brown in colour, about five minutes. Add next five ingredients, turn down heat to medium low and cover. Simmer for about 30 minutes until veggies are soft, stirring occasionally. Then add all spices and stock, turn up heat to medium and low boil another 10 minutes. Remove from burner, add hempseeds and blend all. As a dairy option, serve with a tbsp of sour cream in center of each serving. Serve immediately or refrigerate for next day. This can be frozen as well. Serves six as a starter or four as a meal.

Sumptuous Sides

Holy Guacamole
This will keep in fridge for two days. The trick to this side is that hemp oil keeps the avocado from turning black!

2 tbsp Salba seeds
⅔ cup green onion, finely chopped (approximately 5 small ones)
2 tbsp lime juice or juice of one lime
1 tbsp hemp oil
1½ cups plum tomatoes, diced (approximately 3 large ones)
1 cup fresh cilantro washed and patted dry; once measured, finely chop
4 avocados, diced
¼ tsp garlic powder
½ tsp sea salt
⅓ cup shredded sharp cheddar cheese (optional)

Add first five ingredients together and mix well. Add the rest of the ingredients to tomato mix and gently stir together. Serve with warm whole grain pita pieces.

Hold-the-Mayo Potato Salad

This potato salad is packed with protein and tastes great. Plus it's a great way to ward off the bad fat (mayo) and get reap the benefits of the good ones (EFAs) without losing any of the tasty benefits!

Salad:

> 3 ½ cups pre-boiled and diced yellow potatoes cubed in ½" x ½" pieces, (approximately 5 medium sized ones)
> ½ cup finely chopped green onions (approximately 3 medium ones)
> ¼ cup dill pickles, thinly sliced and diced
> ½ tbsp freshly minced, washed dillweed
> 2 hard boiled eggs (shell off), chopped (optional)
> ¼ tsp ground black pepper
> ¼ tsp ground garlic powder
> ⅛ tsp celery salt
> 1 pinch of ground cumin

Mix the rest of the ingredients together. When well-mixed, slowly add cooked potatoes to mixture. Set aside.

Sauce:

> ⅓ cup commercially-roasted hemp seeds
> ¼ cup dill pickle juice from the jar
> 2 tbsp olive oil
> ½ tsp Dijon mustard
> 1 tbsp water

Blend sauce ingredients in a food processor on high. Drizzle over salad mixture. Mix gently and serve. If you opt for no egg in salad, or like an extra creamy salad, double the sauce recipe. This makes about 4 cups.

Cranberry Quinoa Salad with Tri-Citrus Dressing

This recipe balances sweet and tart flavours and crunchy and soft textures. Plus it's loaded with plant-based proteins and is gluten-free.

Salad:
   1 large apple, chopped
   2 large green onions, finely chopped
   ⅔ cup dried cranberries, finely chopped
   1 cup roasted slivered almonds
   1 cup roasted sesame seeds
   ¾ cup commercially-roasted hemp seeds
   1½ cups cooked quinoa

Dressing:
   2 tbsp maple syrup
   ½ tsp onion powder
   ¼ cup orange juice
   ½ tsp dried ginger
   ½ tsp salt
   Juice of ½ lemon
   Juice of ½ lime
   All cloves from one whole garlic bulb, baked

Combine salad ingredients in a bowl. Blend dressing ingredients and drizzle over salad.

Decadent Delights

So-Free Apple Crisp

This apple crisp is protein-rich with the benefit of oats and is free of butter and refined sugar ... but you would never know it! The coconut oil adds another additional nutritional benefit.

Base:
>   4 cups thinly sliced apples, skin removed (approximately 5 apples)
>   ½ cup raisins or other dried fruit
>   ½ cup maple syrup
>   ⅛ tsp cinnamon
>   ⅛ tsp vanilla

Mix the above together in a 6x10 inch baking dish.

Topping:
>   1 cup oats
>   ⅓ cup unsweetened shredded coconut flakes
>   ½ cup spelt or whole wheat flour
>   ½ cup maple syrup
>   ⅓ cup melted unhydrogenated coconut oil
>   1 tbsp protein powder
>   ¼ tsp cinnamon
>   ¼ tsp vanilla

Preheat oven to 350° F. Mix all topping ingredients together and sprinkle on top of base. Bake for 45 minutes on medium rack. Serve hot or cold.

Sexy Hot Macolate

With the energy-infusing and mood-enhancing properties of Peruvian maca, this one is best reserved for a cold night with your warm honey.

2 cups brown rice milk (or 2% milk)
1 whole (400 g) bar of Macasure Organic chocolate bar
2 tsp of agave syrup
⅛ tsp vanilla extract

Heat brown rice milk (or 2%) on medium/high heat until hot; don't boil. Reduce to low/medium and add all other ingredients. Stir and whisk chocolate until melted. Serve immediately. Makes two big mugs.

Choco-Orange Balls

The dates in this recipe are a great way to get a healthy, sweet taste. These are simple to make and can be easily stored in the fridge or freezer for great protein poppers when needed.

3 cups pitted dates
1 cup orange juice
½ tsp vanilla
2 cups whole cashews or pieces
1 cup commercially-roasted hemp seeds
¾ cup cocoa
½ cup Salba whole seeds

Soak dates, juice and vanilla in a bowl for an hour. In meantime, blend cashews in a food processor until ground and place in a separate bowl. Pulse mix the date mixture in food processor until still a little chunky and not completely smooth. Add date mixture to cashews and add in all other ingredients. Chill mixture in fridge for an hour. Make into quarter size balls and keep in a sealed container in the fridge. Makes about 30 balls.

Choco-Fruit Kebabs

This is a great way to get the nutritional benefits of antioxidants found in both cocoa and fresh fruit. Yes, chocolate can be healthy!

Skewers:
  8 medium-sized strawberries
  8 pieces of pineapple (cut 2x2 inch cube)
  8 pieces of cantaloupe (cut 2x2 inch cube)
  4 wooden skewers
  1 tbsp commercially-roasted hemp seeds

Dip:
  ½ cup commercially-roasted hemp seeds
  3 tbsp warm water
  ¼ cup plus 1 tbsp cocoa powder
  ¼ cup maple syrup or agave nectar
  ½ tsp vanilla
  ¼ tsp cinnamon
  Pinch ground ginger
  Pinch ground nutmeg

Blend roasted hemp seeds and water in a food processor or magic bullet for 1 minute. Add cocoa, maple syrup or agave nectar, vanilla, cinnamon, ginger and nutmeg for another two minutes until creamy consistency.

Clean fruit, pat dry and place on dish. Dip one side of each piece of fruit in the chocolate mixture and then add on to skewer – alternate pineapple/cantaloupe/strawberry. For last strawberry to be skewered (so the first one to be eaten) after dipping in chocolate mixture dip the strawberry tip into the hempseeds for a fun finish. Serve with any leftover dip on the side. Makes four skewers.

Wanna Be a Nut Ball

These are easy to make and are a great nutrient-rich snack. Kids love them and they can be frozen ahead of time and defrosted as needed.

2 tbsp Salba whole seeds
6 tbsp warm water
¼ cup maple syrup
1 tsp vanilla
1 heaping tbsp dried cranberries
6 dried apricots
½ cup walnut pieces
¼ cup oat flakes
1 cup ground blanched almond
½ cup unsweetened shredded coconut
½ cup commercially-roasted hemp seeds
¾ tsp ground cinnamon
¼ tsp ground ginger

Add Salba, water, maple syrup and vanilla together in a bowl and let sit for 15 minutes. In a food processor, blend dried apricots and cranberries with oats and walnut pieces until walnuts are blended and dried fruit is in small pieces. In a mixing bowl, combine Salba and walnut mixture together and then add in all other ingredients. Mix together and make into small quarter sized balls. Put it in a sealed container and keep in the fridge. Makes about 20 balls.

Afterword

Our bodies are our gardens, to which our wills are gardeners.
William Shakespeare, playwright and poet (1564-1616)

We spend so much of our time worrying about the way we look. We make the time to "take care of ourselves" by getting a mani-pedi religiously, with highlights and facials booked weeks in advance and a fortune spent on new clothes. But to truly take care of yourself is to invest in your health and decrease the risk of illness, rather than poisoning the very machine that gives you life itself.

Your body is your temple and you are its only keeper. What you lay at its altar in terms of energy reflects how you worship it and affects how it functions. It is a structure that needs to be constantly maintained and without balancing all three pillars you will ensure its speedy decay. Your temple will eventually topple, as it cannot support the remaining construction.

But embarking upon a HGTV-worthy reno of you does not require drastic measures. In fact, the path to wellness, as you now know, boils down to a few relatively simple principles:
- Increase your consumption of plant-based, nutrient-rich foods like fruits, vegetables, nuts and seeds.
- Don't smoke.
- Maintain a healthy body weight.
- Reduce mental and physical stress.
- Remain physically active.

Among other "details," these are really the basic cornerstones for living a healthier life. But unlike the frazzled immediate-results-based culture in which we live, the achievement of these fundamentals does not have to be instant. In fact, for better results it shouldn't be. Becoming healthier does not have to be overwhelming and should not be mentally or physically stressful.

What does have to take place is a commitment to yourself to be your own caregiver. Don't get locked in your life; instead, embrace it. Take the time to nurture yourself and strive to be a better being every day by taking small but consistent steps. By making these ongoing and positive changes, you will incrementally become healthier. You will slowly look and feel better. You will develop greater physical and mental energy. Over time, you will have greater confidence each passing day, as you strive to be the best you can be. Remember, you do not have to be perfect, other than being perfectly you.[54] Dr. Seuss said it best when he wrote, "Today you are you, that is truer than true. There is no one alive who is you-er than you."

Another famous author, Oscar Wilde, once said, "Experience is the name so many people give to their mistakes." I have to take issue with this approach to life, as I believe the opposite is true: there is no such thing as a mistake. Instead, it is an experience you can draw upon, learn from and share. It is an opportunity to learn about yourself and others around you and to ensure that going forward you will take this new-found knowledge with you. You have earned it.

Like the pride with which girls wear their Brownie badges and boys their Boy Scout achievements, you too must embrace all you have gone through and apply it to the "now." By doing so, the past becomes a well-earned gift that allows for greater knowledge and appreciation of who and where you are, helping you to choose wisely the next path upon which you will embark.

I wish you good health, happiness and lots of laughter in the wonderful time that we all have on this magical planet called Earth. Time is a-ticking, my friend, so get out there, be the better you and make the most of it!

Ann

For more information on living a healthier lifestyle, visit me at www.beabetterbeing.com

Resources & Tips

The following list contains products I've personally tested and use day-to-day when caring for my family and myself.

Hemp

After my foray in law, my husband and I started a health food company. As we researched products, we discovered the wonders of hemp. A sustainable, environmentally-conscious, nutritious and inexpensive crop, we saw a great detail of opportunity to share hemp with families across Canada. All this resulted in our purchase, rebranding and enviro repackaging of Mum's Original products. I use these organic, eco-packaged, nutrient-rich hemp seeds, protein and oil daily as a healthy – yet sneaky – way to add nutrients to family meals.
www.mumsoriginal.com

Salba

For premium white Salvia hispanica L, I choose Salba. Not all Salvia hispanica L is created equal. Research has shown that the white seed has a predisposition to be open when grown to 100 per cent of its potential, which means that your body has the opportunity to absorb all the great nutrients without the need to grind it. Also, the growing condition, including location, is vital, especially as the last three weeks of the 118-day growing cycle are when ALL the antioxidants and a whopping one-third of the omegas are actually formed. Many non-food Salvia hispanica L growers do not wait for the last trimester to harvest their grain, as it is still valuable as feed when harvested earlier and the risk of damage by rain or other crop failure is reduced. There are very few growers around the world who grow pure white Salvia hispanica L for food so you want to opt only for the premium, heirloom white Salvia hispanica L in order to reap the maximum benefits that this incredible whole food has to offer. My intricate knowledge of this amazing crop was learned in the process of owning and operating the Source Salba company with my husband.
www.sourcesalba.com

Beans

Although I prefer to buy dried beans and soak them to increase the nutritional value, sometimes I run out of time. Then, I turn to canned beans from Eden Foods. They offer premium organic products that are locally-sourced and they work directly with growers and co-packers with similar environmental focuses.

www.edenfoods.com

Coconut Oil

Coconut oil is so delicious and healthy. I have found a number of excellent lines, but I think my favourite is the Wilderness Family Naturals line. These people truly live the life, know their coconuts and offer up tasty and organic coconut oil.

www.wildernessfamilynaturals.com

Condiments

A great alternative to soya sauce or tamari is Braggs Liquid Amino. With 16 amino acids, it is an excellent way to add a splash of flavour to any stir-fries, soups or stews. They also have an excellent apple cider vinegar, which helps to restabilize pH levels.

www.bragg.com

Co-ops

This is one of the best-kept secrets for affordably outfitting your family with organic products. I buy all my frozen and canned products through a local food co-op. I cannot say enough about how easy and cheap it is to use! You set yourself up as a "store" or buying club, get together with friends or family, and make a larger grocery order to get the benefit of cheaper prices. Also, I only have to order groceries once every four to eight weeks and they are delivered right to the front door.

www.planetfriendly.net

www.localharvest.org

Dairy Products

When I do need a fix of butter or cheese, I turn to L'Ancêtre Cheese Factory. They are a Quebec company founded by a group of ten milk

producers with a different vision than those in conventional agriculture: conscientious farming and animal treatment. I find that when I need that dairy treat their organic cheese is the best and richest-tasting.
www.fromagerieancetre.com

Ethnic Ingredients

My favourite chickpea and specialty flours and spices come from a Canadian company called ShaShi Foods (King of Spices). They are a family-run business that custom grinds and blends their spices, herbs, seasoning blends and specialty flours. I find their products to be super fresh, as they blend them all themselves and source the raw materials from around the world. They also offer the Pataks line of curries which is a great starting point for stews and curry dishes! For organic spices, which are a little more expensive, I opt for the Frontier Natural Products Co-op line of dried herbs and spices.
www.shashi.ca
www.frontiercoop.com

Farmers' Markets

A great local resource to find organic produce is your local farmers' market. I feel better knowing my produce was grown only a few minutes away and I'm supporting local business. To find your local farmers' market, check out the available online databases.
www.planetfriendly.net
www.localharvest.org

Household Cleaning

For cleaning, I like to use the Nellie's All-Natural Products. Not only are their products excellent and eco-friendly, but their reusable and recyclable tins are a happy edition to my kitchen storage area. Nature Clean is also an excellent line of household cleaning supplies with incredible natural and effective products to keep your home clean.
www.nelliesallnatural.com
www.naturecleanliving.com

Maca

When I need an energy boost, I add a spoonful of maca powder to my morning smoothie. Maca is a nutritious root vegetable from Peru that regulates and restores hormonal balance, helps reduce stress, improves sexual function and increases energy. MacaSure offers high quality, fairly-traded maca in powder and capsules. They also have a delicious dark chocolate bar with a full serving of maca.

www.macasure.com

Milk Alternatives

I try to limit the amount of cow milk I use, as it can be an allergen and our son has the early signs of asthma. For milk alternatives, I use Natur-a rice milks by Nutrisoya. I like this company because they have certified organic foods, use healthy farming and production practices and incorporate environmental-protection processes and waste by-product recycling. For another non-dairy alternative, I like to add in almond milk, which I get from Almond Fresh.

www.nutrisoya.com

www.earthsown.ca

Nut Butters

For my nut butters, I try to get them freshly pureed at my local health food store, but if I have no time I reach for MaraNatha nut butters. They have a range of organic and natural nut and seed butters that are free of trans fats, hydrogenated oils and preservatives with an organic and salt-free line of butters.

www.maranathafoods.com

Nutritional Supplements

The line of plant-based, whole foods, created by professional triathlete and vegan Brendan Brazier includes smoothie mixes, energy and snack bars. We regularly add Vega Smoothie Infusion to nutritious goodies for the kids, as it is a great way to add extra nutrition. For a green boost to my smoothies every morning I like to use Amazing Grass Green SuperFood. Their Berry Flavour is excellent and my children even love it.

www.amazinggrass.com

www.myvega.com

Psuedograins

For quinoa and amaranth, I use GoGoQuino organic and gluten-free products made from grains grown in Bolivia. Their fair-trade products also help to ensure sustainable development through the Bolivian co-ops with which they work.
www.gogoquinoa.com

Rice

For rice that is an excellent accompaniment to the many bean dishes I make, the one I love the most is Lundberg. They specialize in organic and whole grain rice products and have so many options to explore. I support them as they focus on sustainable growing practices and are family-owned.
www.lundberg.com

Snack Food

When I want that salty snack, I reach for the organic Hippy Chips made with whole grains and Skeet & Ike's flavourful organic popcorn. You can't beat them when you crave tasty crunchy treats!
www.skeetandikes.com
www.hippychips.com

Soy

Although I don't eat a lot of soy, if I need a soy fix I always buy the Sol-Cuisine brand of Tofu and various food products. All their soy is locally-grown and non-GMO with tier 1 production processes. Unlike many other soy production facilities located overseas, there is no use of aluminum vats in the production process and Sol-Cuisine ensures sustainable growing practices.
www.solcuisine.com

Toiletries

For excellent skin, hair and facial care products that are paraben- and toxin-free, I use the Green Beaver line, a Canadian company that is family-run and produces all their products without chemical preservatives, fragrances or dyes.
www.greenbeaver.com

Aubrey Organics saved my skin cancer anxiety with their incredibly effective and natural sun care line of products. With no parabens or other toxins, I can properly protect my children's skin without worry. www.aubrey-organics.com

I also have a huge amount of respect for the Annemarie Borlind line of skin cream. They use only natural, cruelty-free ingredients and extract their ingredients with organic cultivation. They truly walk the talk with their incredible sustainable farming practices and are involved in every aspect of the products' raw material, production and packaging. www.borlind.com

Zuzu Luxe line of cosmetics is incredible. After throwing out all my makeup I sampled many lines and theirs is one of my favourites. Their lipstick is superior in colour and staying power, their blush is phenomenal and their lip and eyeliners are better and cheaper than the toxic designer ones I used to buy. www.gabrielcosmeticsinc.com

Toothpaste

Kiss My Face toothpaste is the best I have tried. They are an independent natural and organic-focused company that makes a healthy and effective toothpaste our whole family loves. Green Beaver also makes a very clean toothpaste with many kid-friendly flavours. www.kissmyface.com www.greenbeaver.com

Vitamins

During the winter months or when I'm feeling run down, I opt for a vitamin C boost with the Emergen-C vitamin C drink mixes. I can also effectively get vitamin C and multivitamins into my kids when their systems are low with the easy-to-use Emergen-C Kidz line. www.emergenc.com

Water Filter

When I lived in the city and did not have my current fresh well water, I used the Santevia Enhanced Water System to naturally filter the extensive chemicals out of our water. It was simple to use and the water tasted great. Plus, we got rid of our eco-unfriendly water jugs.

www.santevia.com

References

1   CIHR Research Chair in Obesity. Retrieved from: http://obesity.ulaval.ca/obesity/generalities/prevalence.php

2   CDC/NCHS, Health, United States, 2006. http://win.niddk.nih.gov/statistics/

3   The NPD Group Inc. "NPD Finds Moms' Eating Habits and Nutritional Knowledge Influences What Their Kids Eat." October 19, 2009.

4   Breast milk is approximately 50 per cent fat as babies need this to build their brains.

5   Thuc T Le, Terry B Huff, and Ji-Xin Cheng, Coherent anti-Stokes Raman scattering imaging of lipids in cancer metastasis, BMC Cancer. 2009; 9:42 .

6   Belch, JJF, Muir, A. N-6 and n-3 essential fatty acids in rheumatoid arthritis and other rheumatic conditions. Proceedings of the Nutrition Society (1998), 57,563-569; Zurier, RB, Rossetti, RG, Jacobson EW, et al. Gamma-linolenic acid treatment of rheumatoid arthritis. A randomized placebo-controlled trial. Arthritis Rheum. 1996 Nov; 39(11): 1808-17; Levelthal, LJ, Boyce, EG, Zurier, RB. Treatment of rheunatois arthritis with gammalinolenic acid. Ann Intern Med. 1993 Nov1; 119(9): 867-73. 1993; Callaway J, Schwab U, Harvima I, et al. Efficacy of dietary hempseed oil in patients with atopic dermatitis. J Dermatolog Treat. 2005; Surette, ME, Stull, D, Lindeman, J. The impact of a medical food containing gammalinolenic and eicosapentaennoic acids on asthma management and the quality of life of adult asthma patients. Curr Med Opin. 2008 Feb; 24(2): 559-67; 31. Menendez,JA, Lupu, R. RESPONSE: Re: Effect of gamma-Linolenic Acid on the Transcriptional Activity of the Her-2/neu (erbB-2) Oncogene. Journal of the National Cancer Institute 2006 98(10):718-720.

7   W.C. Willett, M.J. Stampfer, J.E. Mason, G.A. Colditz, F.E. Speizer, B.A. Rosner, L.A. Sampson, C.H. Hennekes, Intake of trans fatty acids and risk of coronary heart disease among women, Lancet 341, 581-585 (1993). F.B. Hu, M.J. Stampfer, J.E. Manson, E. Rimm, G.A. Colditz, B.A. Rosner, C.H. Hennekens, W.C. Willett, Dietary Fat Intake and the Risk of Coronary Heart Disease in Women, New England Journal of Medicine 337, 1491-1499 (1997). K. Hayakawa, Y.Y. Linko, P. Linko, The role of trans fatty acids in human nutrition, Journal of Lipid Science and Technology 102, 419-425 (2000).

8   Health effects of oxidized heated oils, Martin Grootveld, Christopher J.L. Silwood, Paul Addis And Rew Claxson, Bartolomé Bonet Serra And Marta Viana, 2001, Foodservice Research International 13(1):41-55.

9   Health Effects Of Oxidized Heated Oils, Martin Grootveld, Christopher J.L. Silwood, Paul Addis And Rew Claxson, Bartolomé Bonet Serra And Marta Viana, 2001, Foodservice Research International 13(1):41-55.

10   11 Table information adapted from Smoke Point of Various Fats, by Michael Chu, www.cookingforengineers.com.

Leah B. Sansbury, Kay Wanke, Paul S. Albert, Lisa Kahle,Arthur Schatzkin, Elaine Lanza andthe Polyp Prevention Trial Study Group, "The Effect of Strict Adherence to a High-Fiber, High-Fruit and -Vegetable, and Low-Fat Eating Pattern on Adenoma Recurrence", American Journal of Epidemiology 2009 170(5):576-584

12   Note that the recommended fibre intake for children differs from that of adults and can be calculated

by adding five grams of fibre to the child's age in years.

13   World Cancer Research Fund's report, Food, Nutrition, Physical Activity and the Prevention of Cancer: a Global Perspective (2007).

14   Brazier, Brendan. The Thrive Diet, Penguin Publishing, 2007 p.71.

15   World Health Organization, Cardiovascular Disease, Fact sheet N°317, updated September 2009

16   World Health Organization, Cardiovascular Disease, Fact sheet N°317, updated September 2009

17   American Heart Association.

18   New British Heart Foundation's research from Imperial College London.

19   Ellen Tattleman, Health Effects of Garlic, American Family Physician, July 2005.

20   H. Ting et al., Journal of Clinical Investigation 97:22-8, Jan. 1996.

21   M. Laidlaw and B. Holub, Effects of supplementation with fish oil–derived n-3 fatty acids and gamma-linolenic acid on circulating plasma lipids and fatty acid profiles in women, American Journal of Clinical Nutrition, Vol. 77, No. 1, 37-42, January 2003.

22   National Cancer Institute, Retrieved from http://www.cancer.gov/cancertopics/factsheet/Risk/obesity

23   Allen NE, Beral V, Casabonne D, et al. Moderate alcohol intake and cancer incidence in women. Journal of the National Cancer Institute. 2009; 101: 296-305

24   National Cancer Institute.

25   Cattlemen's Beef Board & National Cattlemen's Beef Association (2003). Heterocyclic amines in food and their implications for health. Retrieved from http://www.beefnutrition.org. Salmon, C.P., Knize, M.G., Panteleakos, F.N., et al., (2000). Minimization of Heterocyclic Amines and Thermal Inactivation of Escheri salvia hispanica L coli in Fried Ground Beef. Journal of the National Cancer Institute. 92(21), 1773-1778. United States Department of Health and Human Services, Public Health (1995). Toxicological Profile for Polycyclic Aromatic Hydrocarbons. Retrieved from http://www.atsdr.cdc.gov/toxprofiles/tp69.pdf

26   Nerurkar, P., Le Marchand, L., & Cooney, R. (1999). Effects of marinating with Asian marinades or western barbecue sauce on PhIP and MeIQx formation in barbecued beef.Nutrition and Cancer, 34 (2), 147-152. Salmon, C.P., Knize, M.G., & Felton, J.S. (1997). Effects of Marinating on Heterocyclic Amine Carcinogen Formation in Grilled Chicken. Food and Chemical Technology, 35, 433-441.

27   National Cancer Institute.

28   United States Environmental Protection Agency, Carcinogenicity Assessment for Lifetime Exposure.

29   Cancer Research UK

30   Akinori Yanaka, Jed W. Fahey, Atsushi Fukumoto, Mari Nakayama, Souta Inoue, Songhua Zhang, Masafumi Tauchi, Hideo Suzuki, Ichinosuke Hyodoand Masayuki Yamamoto, Dietary Sulforaphane-Rich Broccoli Sprouts Reduce Colonization and Attenuate Gastritis in Helicobacter pylori–

Infected Mice and Humans. Cancer Prevention Research 2, 353, April 1, 2009.

31   Natural Medicines Comprehensive Database: "Ovarian Cancer"; Jellin. J. (Editor); Updated June 13, 2008.

32   F. Kenny, S. Pinder, I. Ellis, R. Bryce, J. Hartley, J. Robertson, Gamma linolenic acid with tamoxifen as primary therapy in breast cancer, European Journal of Cancer, Volume 34, Issue null, Pages S18-S19

33   Menendez, J.A., Lupu R. Response: Re: Effect of Gamma-Linolenic Acid on the Transcriptional Activity of the Her-2/neu (erbB-2) Oncogene. Journal of the National Cancer Institute , 2006 98(10): 718-720.

34   Bingham SA, Day NE, Luben R, Ferrari P, Slimani N, Norat T, Clavel-Chapelon F, Kesse E, Nieters A, Boeing H, Tjønneland A, Overvad K, Martinez C, Dorronsoro M, Gonzalez CA, Key TJ, Trichopoulou A, Naska A, Vineis P, Tumino R, Krogh V, Bueno-de-Mesquita HB,Peeters PH, Berglund G, Hallmans G, Lund E, Skeie G, Kaaks R, Riboli E; European Prospective Investigation into Cancer and Nutrition. "Dietary fibre in food and protection against colorectal cancer in the European Prospective Investigation into Cancer and Nutrition (EPIC): an observational study". Lancet. 2003 May 3;361(9368):1496-501

35   Albaines, D. et al. Alpha-Tocopheral and beta-carotene supplements and lung cancer incidence in the alpha-tocopherol, beta-carotene cancer prevention study: effects of baseline characteristics and study compliance. Journal of the National Cancer Institute. 1996. 88(21):1560-70. Satia, J. et al. Long-term Use of B-Carotene, Retinol, Lycopene and Lutein Supplements and Lung Cancer Risk: Results From the VITamins And Lifestyle (VITAL) Study. American Journal of Epidemiology. 2009. 164(7):815-828.

36   The Link between Diabetes and Cardio Vascular Disease, U.S. Department of Health and Human Services' National Diabetes Education, February 2007

37   The Link between Diabetes and Cardio Vascular Disease, U.S. Department of Health and Human Services' National Diabetes Education, February 2007.

38   Nathan DM, Cleary PA, Backlund JY, et al. Intensive diabetes treatment and cardiovascular disease in patients with type 1 diabetes. N Engl J Med. Dec 22 2005⊠353(25):26432653.

39   National Institute of Diabetes and Digestive and Kidney Diseases. National diabetes statistics fact sheet: general information and national estimates on diabetes in the United States, 2005. Bethesda, MD: U.S. Department of Health and Human Services, National Institutes of Health⊠ 2005.

40   The Link between Diabetes and Cardio Vascular Disease, U.S. Department of Health and Human S ervices' National Diabetes Education, February 2007.

41   University of Toronto, Diabetes Care. November, 2007.

42   Neilsen Global Online. "Neilsen: Diet and Eating: A Canadian Perspective". The Neilsen Company, November 2008.

43   Marketdata Enterprises, 2007, study of American weight loss industry in 2006.

44   Mann T, Tomiyama AJ, Westling E, Lew AM, Samuels B, Chatman J. "Medicare's Search for Effective Obesity Treatments: Diets Are Not the Answer." Am Psychol. 2007 Apr;62(3):220-33.

45   For an intense lesson on breathing techniques for stress reduction, try the free Oceanic Breathing lesson at http://foreverlivinghealth.com/sc-ob.html.

46   Rena R Wing, James O Hill. "Successful Weight Loss Maintenance". Annual Review Of Nutrition, 2001, Jul, 21 323-341.

47   If your actions are harming or potentially harming any of God's creatures, or are putting your personal safety at risk then put this book down now, grab the yellow pages and call one of the many organizations out there for help. Physical addictions to drugs and alcohol or addictions that prevent you from living your life in a productive way are extreme levels of dependency usually requiring professional help, so if this is you, get it. If you seek help, you shall find it.

48   http://www.cmha.ca

49   http://www.cmha.ca

50   I am picking on mother-in-laws here as humorous relief. Mine is lovely and we get along really well. She has never stolen a wagon wheel from me.

51   Brazier, Brendan. Penguin Publishing, The Thrive Diet, 2007. Page 14.

52   Brazier, Brendan. Penguin Publishing, The Thrive Diet, 2007. Page 71.

53   Alice Domar Ph.D.Harvard Medical School.

54   I give full credit to this great quote to my wise friend, Peter Smyth.

Notes to Self

Notes to Self

Notes to Self